Progress in Hormone Biochemistry and Pharmacology

Volume 1

MICHAEL BRIGGS
Professor of Human Biology
Dean of Science
Deakin University, Belmont
Victoria, Australia.

ALAN CORBIN
Head, Endocrinology
Research and Development Department
Wyeth Laboratories Inc.
Philadelphia, Pennsylvania.

Eden Press
MEDICAL & SCIENTIFIC PUBLISHERS

MTP PRESS LIMITED · LANCASTER · ENGLAND
International Medical Publishers

ISBN-13: 978-94-011-7714-6 e-ISBN-13: 978-94-011-7712-2

DOI: 10.1007/ 978-94-011-7712-2

Softcover reprint of the hardcover 1st edition 1980

Published simultaneously in Canada by
Eden Press Inc., Suite 10, 245 Victoria Avenue, Westmount, Quebec H3Z 2M6

in the United States of America by
Eden Medical Research Inc., PO Box 51, St. Albans, VT 05478

and in the United Kingdom and Europe by
MTP Press Limited, Falcon House, Cable Street, Lancaster, England

Contributors

Michael J. Antonaccio, Squibb Institute for Medical Research, PO Box 4000, Princeton, NJ 08540

Frederick J. Bex, Endocrinology Section, Wyeth Laboratories Inc., Box 8299, Philadelphia, PA 19101

Audrey S. Bingel, Department of Pharmacognasy and Pharmacology, College of Pharmacy, University of Illinois at the Medical Center, Box 6998, Chicago, IL 60680

Alan Corbin, Endocrinology Section, Wyeth Laboratories Inc., Box 8299, Philadelphia, PA 19101

Norman R. Farnsworth, Department of Pharmacognasy and Pharmacology, College of Pharmacy, University of Illinois at the Medical Center, Box 6998, Chicago, IL 60680

John E. Gerich, Endocrine Research Unit, Departments of Medicine and Physiology, Mayo Clinic and Mayo Medical School, Rochester, MN 55901

Zola P. Horovitz, Squibb Institute for Medical Research, PO Box 4000, Princeton, NJ 08540

Bernard Rubin, Squibb Institute for Medical Research, PO Box 4000, Princeton, NJ 08540

Editorial

Endocrinology is a scientific discovery of the 20th century. Progress in the understanding of hormone actions at the biochemical level, and the development of this knowledge into pharmaceutical products for use in human and veterinary medicine, has grown at an exponential rate in recent years. It is hard to believe that the chemical nature of the steroid hormones was unknown until the 1930's, that metabolic conversion of vitamin D to circulating hormones was only discovered in 1966, that the very existence of human prolactin was debated up to 10 years ago, and that the hypothalamic releasing hormones were identified and purified less than 20 years ago. The discovery of potent locally-acting substances of short biological half-life, such as cyclic-AMP, prostaglandins, and thromboxanes has added a new dimension to endocrinology. Textbooks more than five years old are not just out of date: they are frankly misleading.

Almost every discovery in endocrine biochemistry has led to new pharmaceutical products, many of which have revolutionised our lives. Obvious examples are insulin for diabetics, corticosteroids for numerous inflammatory diseases, sex hormones for contraception, prostaglandins for the termination of pregnancy, and β-blocking drugs for the treatment of hypertension. There is presently intense activity with releasing hormones, which may offer a safer approach to fertility control in both men and women.

It is with this background that the idea of a series of review publications was born. The Editors' intention is to identify workers in rapidly developing areas of endocrine biochemistry or pharmacology and to invite them to prepare a definitive presentation of their field. By using camera-ready manuscripts, the volume will be produced and released in three to four months. Initially, it is hoped to produce a volume of five or six reviews every two years. No attempt will be made to cover all areas of endocrinology, just those where progress is occurring at a rapid rate.

The Editors would be interested to receive suggestions of possible topics to be covered in future volumes.

M.H.B.
A.C.

CONTENTS

1 **The Renin-Angiotensin System, Converting Enzyme Inhibition, and Antihypertensive Therapy** 1
B. Rubin, M.J. Antonaccio & Z.P. Horovitz

The Renin-Angiotensin-Aldosterone System and the Kallikrein-Kinin-Prostaglandin System ...3; Converting Enzyme Inhibition: Biochemical and Pharmacological Studies ...8; Effects on Blood Pressure ...16; Antihypertensive Actions in Man ...24; Hemodynamics ...29; Endocrinological Effects ...30; Water, Sodium, and Potassium ...32; Congestive Heart Failure ...32; Hemorrhagic Shock ...33; Mechanism of Action ...33; References ...41

2 **The Pharmacology and Potential Clinical Applications of Somatostatin and its Analogues** 55
J.E. Gerich

Background ...56; General Distributions and Actions ...58; Mechanism of Action ...72; Metabolism ...77; Physiologic Role of Endogenous Somatostatin ...77; Regulation of Pancreatic Somatostatin Secretion in Vitro ...79; Therapeutic Potential of Somatostatin in Diabetes Mellitus and other Disorders ...89; Structure-Activity Relationships: Analogues ...93; References ...99

3 **Botanical Sources of Fertility Regulating Agents: Chemistry and Pharmacology** 149

A.S. Bingel & N.R. Farnsworth

Introduction ...150; Estrogenic Plants ...151; Fertility Control in the Female ...156; Vaginal Contraceptives ...179; Fertility Control in the Male ...184; Discussion ...193; References ...205

4 **Luteinizing Hormone Releasing Hormone and Analogues: Conceptive and Contraceptive Potential** 227

A. Corbin & F.J. Bex

Introduction ...228; Conceptive Aspects ...229; Contraceptive Aspects ...236; Conclusions ...273; References ...277

Index 299

PROGRESS IN
HORMONE BIOCHEMISTRY AND PHARMACOLOGY

1. THE RENIN-ANGIOTENSIN SYSTEM, CONVERTING ENZYME INHIBITION, AND ANTIHYPERTENSIVE THERAPY

B. Rubin, M.J. Antonaccio & Z.P. Horovitz

1. **The Renin-Angiotensin-Aldosterone System and the Kallikrein-Kinin-Prostaglandin System...3**
   A. General Functional Aspects 3; B. Historical: Biochemical, Physiological, and Pharmacological Background 6.

2. **Converting Enzyme Inhibition: Biochemical and Pharmacological Studies...8**
   A. Inhibitory Peptides from Snake Venom (teprotide, etc.) 8; B. Design of Non-Peptidic Site-Directed Inhibitory Compounds (captopril) 9; C. *In Vitro* Inhibition of Converting Enzyme 11; D. *In Vivo* Inhibition of Converting Enzyme 12.

3. **Effects on Blood Pressure...16**
   A. Normotensive Models 16; B. Renal Hypertension 16; C. One Kidney, One Clip Hypertension 19; D. Genetic (Spontaneous) Hypertension 21; E. DOCA-Salt Hypertension 24; F. Other Models of Hypertension 24.

4. **Antihypertensive Actions in Man...24**

5. **Hemodynamics...29**
   A. Animal Studies 29; B. Human Studies 30.

6. **Endocrinological Effects...30**
   A. Renin Activity 30; B. Angiotensin I, Angiotensin II, Aldosterone, and Bradykinin 31.

(Continued overleaf)

7. **Water, Sodium, and Potassium...32**

8. **Congestive Heart Failure...32**

9. **Hemorrhagic Shock...33**

10. **Mechanism of Action...33**
A. Arterial Wall Renin 35; B. Bradykinin Accumulation 36;
C. Prostaglandin Release 38; D. Kidneys and Adrenal Glands 38;
E. Sodium and Water Excretion 39.

References...41

In the past 80 years, the renin-angiotensin-aldosterone system, the kallikrein-kinin-prostaglandin system, and the role of the angiotensin-converting enzyme have been undergoing ever-increasing investigation in the pathogenesis of hypertension and in related cardiovascular disorders. Much insight has been obtained, but, controversial findings in some areas give further promise of even more biochemical and physiological, and pharmacological studies and analyses in animals and in man.

The major objectives of this review are (1) to briefly examine the historical development of the biochemical, physiological characteristics and current concepts of the renin-angiotensin-aldosterone and of the kallikrein-kinin-prostaglandin systems as well as those of the actions of the angiotensin-converting enzyme (ACE), (2) to indicate how malfunction(s) of any of these several systems can be contributory or important factors in the pathophysiology of hypertensive, renal, or other cardiovascular disorders, (3) to present the evidence which (a) demonstrates, both experimentally and clinically, the antihypertensive and other therapeutic effectiveness of specific and potent inhibitors of ACE such as the nonapeptide teprotide[1,2] and the non-peptidic compound captopril[3] (b) indicates or suggests the mechanism(s) of action of such compounds.

1. The Renin Angiotensin-Aldosterone System and the Kallikrein-Kinin-Prostaglandin System

A. General Functional Aspects

The renin-angiotensin-aldosterone and the kallikrein-kinin-prostaglandin systems comprise homeostatic cardiovascular mechanisms (Fig. 1). Factors that lower blood volume, renal perfusion or plasma Na+ concentration tend to stimulate the secretion of the endopeptidase renin from the juxtaglomerular apparatus of the kidney. Factors that act in the opposite direction tend to

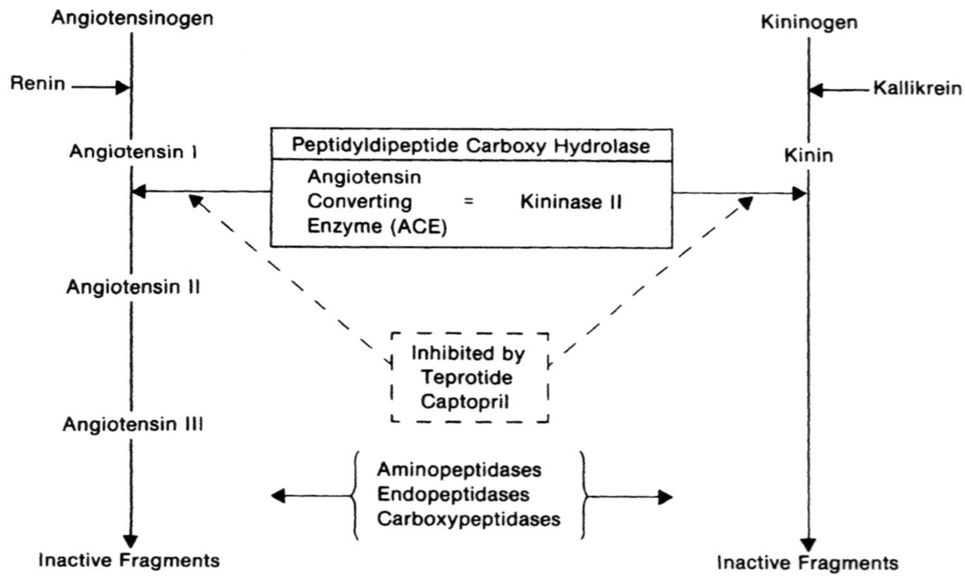

FIG. 1: Outline of renin-angiotensin system and kallikrein-kinin system and of the roles played by peptidyldipeptide carboxy hydrolase. Captopril, as well as teprotide, inhibits this enzyme and thereby reduces cleavage of C-terminal dipeptides from angiotensin I as well as from bradykinin. *(Reprinted with permission from Cushman DW, Cheung HS, Sabo EF and Ondetti MA. Design of potent competitive inhibitors of angiotensin-converting enzyme. Carboxyalkanoyl and mercaptoalkanoyl amino acids. Biochemistry 16: 5484-5491, 1977. Copyright by the American Chemical Society.)*

inhibit secretion of renin. An increase in renin production increases formation of angiotensin I (AI) from angiotensinogen, a blood glycoprotein. AI, a decapeptide which is relatively inactive, is converted by angiotensin converting enzyme (ACE), a carboxypeptidase, to the octapeptide angiotensin II (AII). AII causes vasoconstriction and stimulates aldosterone secretion which in turn leads to Na+ retention, increases in blood volume and increase in blood pressure. The increases in blood pressure and/or plasma Na+ tend to inhibit renin release; as an ensuing Na+ depletion develops, blood volume falls and blood pressure declines. With the decrease in blood pressure and volume the cycle is then reactivated.[4-8]

On the other hand, the kallikrein-kinin-prostaglandin system tends to promote vasodilation and lowering of blood pressure, and in most animals, to increase renal blood flow, diuresis and natriuresis. Kallikreins (or kininogenases) are plasma and tissue enzymes (pancreatic, salivary, renal, etc.) which act upon plasma globulins (kininogens) to release kinins which are polypeptides. Two of the most widely studied kinins are the nonapeptide bradykinin and the decapeptide lysyl-bradykinin (kallidin).[9-13]

ACE, an exopeptidase obtained from lung, plasma or serum, or kidney of several animal species has been usually reported to be a glycoprotein with a single polypeptide chain, a polysaccharide residue, and one zinc atom per molecule; its molecular weight is at least 129,000 (see review by Cushman and Ondetti[14]). ACE and kininase II are apparently the same peptidyl-dipeptide carboxy hydrolase (E.C.3.4.15.1).[15-17]

Inhibitors of the enzymes ACE or kininase II can reduce the formation of AII from AI and inhibit the degradation of bradykinin (Fig. 1). Thus, such inhibitors can strongly influence the renin-angiotensin-aldosterone and the kallikrein-kinin-prostaglandin systems with the potential net results of lowering blood pressure, promoting natriuresis, decreasing aldosterone secretion, increasing intrarenal effects of bradykinin and of other autacoids such as the prostaglandins.

In considering here the development of inhibitors of angiotensin-converting enzyme or kininase II, and the use of such inhibitors as antihypertensive agents, a brief review of the major developments of past decades concerning the renin-angiotensin-aldosterone and the kallikrein-kinin-prostaglandin systems is warranted. These developments have laid the groundwork for more recent and current studies in this field. Limitation of space, however, permits citing the work of only some of the key investigators. Many reviews dealing more comprehensively with the history and current status of this subject are available.[4-24]

1B. Historical: Biochemical, Physiological, and Pharmacological Background

The story of the renin-angiotensin system has its beginnings in 1898 when Tigerstedt and Bergman[25] found that extracts of the kidney contained a pressor substance which they called renin. By 1934, Goldblatt *et al.*[26] had found pressor activity in renal venous blood after constriction of the renal artery; this activity was attributed to renin. In 1939-1940 Braun-Menéndez *et al.*[27] and Page and Helmer[28] found that renin was an enzyme in the cascade that resulted in the formation of a pressor peptide from a plasma protein substrate. This pressor peptide was renamed angiotensin in 1958 by Braun-Menéndez and Page[29] (after having been previously known as angiotonin and hypertensin); also, the plasma substrate was named angiotensinogen. In 1954, Skeggs *et al.*[30] reported that angiotensin was a mixture of the relatively inactive decapeptide angiotensin I (AI) and the very active octapeptide angiotensin II (AII). AII was then shown to originate from the inactive AI by the action of angiotensin converting enzyme discovered in plasma by the same investigators.[31] ACE is a peptidyldipeptide carboxy hydrolase which cleaves the dipeptide histidyl-leucine from the carboxyl end of AI.[15-17] In 1956-7, Elliott and Peart[32] and Skeggs et al.[33] described the amino acid sequence of angiotensin II, which was then synthesized by Schwyzer et al.,[34] and Bumpus et al.[35] During 1958-1962, a series of key studies by Carpenter et al.,[36] Genest et al.,[37] Gross,[38] Laragh[39] and Mulrow et al.[40] revealed that the renin-angiotensin system was implicated in electrolyte balance and in the regulation of aldosterone secretion by the adrenal cortex. Thus, in addition to vasoconstrictor actions, the renin-angiotensin system served as a mechanism to stimulate aldosterone secretion and thereby acted to conserve sodium and maintain blood volume. In 1967, Ng and Vane[41] showed that the lung was the principal site of conversion of AI to AII. More recently, Blair-west et al.[42] and Goodfriend and Peach[43] reported that AII may be acted upon by an aminopeptidase to form the heptapeptide des-Asp^1-AII, sometimes referred to as angiotensin III (AIII). AIII has been found to be somewhat less pressor than AII and was previously believed to be about equally as active as AII in releasing aldosterone from the adrenal cortex. The latter finding has been recently questioned by McCaa.[44] AI, AII and AIII are subject to the action of various aminopeptidases, endopeptidases and/or carboxypeptidases, eventually leading to inactive fragments.[7,14-17,20]

In a series of papers during 1926 to 1948 (as reviewed by Werle[45]), Frey, Kraut and Werle and their associates discovered and described the vasodepressor actions of a new principle found in urine, plasma, kidney, and in some glands (such as the pancreas); this principle was designated as kallikrein, now also known as kininogenase.[18,19,46,47] Plasma kallikrein is a proteolytic enzyme which acts upon an inactive precursor present in a plasma globulin fraction (kininogen) to form active kinin peptides such as bradykinin. It was apparent to Werle that kinins could be rapidly inactivated by peptidases, now known as kininases. In 1949, Rocha e Silva, Beraldo and Rosenfeld[48] found and characterized the first kinin and named it bradykinin; they obtained bradykinin by treating plasma globulin with certain snake venoms or trypsin. Bradykinin lowers blood pressure and slowly contracts isolated gut tissue. In 1960 the structure of bradykinin was elucidated by the combined efforts of Elliott et al.[49] and by Boissonnas and associates;[50] the latter group described the first synthesis of this kinin. Bradykinin may also be formed from lysylbradykinin (kallidin) by the action of plasma aminopeptidase; the two peptides are cleaved from a common kininogen precursor by kallikrein. Kallidin is formed by glandular, urinary, and renal kallikreins acting upon kallidinogen. Between 1966 and 1976, Erdös and associates[15-18] marshalled evidence that ACE and kininase II were identical. Kininase II cleaves and inactivates bradykinin, primarily by hydrolytic removal of its carboxyl terminal phenylalanyl-arginine dipeptide.[51]

2. Converting Enzyme Inhibition: Biochemical and Pharmacological studies.

A. Inhibitory Peptides from Snake Venom (teprotide, etc.)

In 1965, Ferreira[52] described the presence in the venom of the Brazilian "arrowhead" viper, *Bothrops jararaca*, of compounds capable of potentiating the activity of bradykinin and which he designated as bradykinin-potentiating factor (BPF). Three years later, Bakhle[53] reported that BPF was also a potent inhibitor of ACE. Ferreira et al.[54,55] in 1970 isolated 9 bradykinin-potentiating peptides from the venom of *B. jararaca* and defined the amino acid sequence of one of the 9 peptides, a pentapeptide, later called BPP_{5a}. BPP_{5a} was synthesized by Stewart et al.[56] in 1971. Synthetic BPP_{5a} (<Glu-Lys-Trp-Ala-Pro) and the other peptide fractions were all capable of inhibiting ACE.[2,56,57] In 1971, Ondetti et al.[1] described the isolation and structure of 6 ACE inhibitory peptides from *B. jararaca* venom. These 6 peptides

ranged in size from nonapeptide to tridecapeptide and their proposed sequences were confirmed by synthesis. Five of the 6 peptides are probably identical to those isolated by Ferreira and associates. Their inhibitory properties on rabbit lung ACE, including those of the nonapeptide teprotide (SQ 20,881, BPP_{9a}), were described by Cheung and Cushman in 1973.[2] The nonapeptide teprotide (<Glu-Trp-Pro-Arg-Pro-Gln-Ile-Pro-Pro), like other peptides in the venom, augmented the vasodepressor and other biological activities of bradykinin.[58,59] Inhibition of ACE has also been reported for peptides isolated by Kato and Suzuki[60] from the venom of the Asia pit viper (*Agkistrodon halys blomhoffii*).

Teprotide has been studied extensively *in vitro*[2,51,59,61] and *in vivo* including normotensive and experimentally hypertensive animal models[58,62-64] as well as in normotensive, renovascular and essential hypertensive man.[65-68] Teprotide has a longer duration of action *in vivo* than does BPP_{5a} with reference to specifically inhibiting the pressor action of AI or augmenting the depressor action of exogenous bradykinin.[46,58,61,69] Teprotide's lack of oral activity has been its major limitation; hence, practically all preclinical and clinical studies with teprotide indicating its efficacy as an inhibitor of ACE or kininase II (Fig. 2) and as an antihypertensive agent have been conducted by parenteral (often intravenous) routes of dosage, in contrast with most of the studies conducted with the orally effective inhibitor, captopril.

2B. Design of Non-Peptidic Site-Directed Inhibitory Compounds (captopril)

Captopril was developed from a program of rational chemical design that made use of a hypothetical model of the active site of ACE as the basis for synthesis of compounds with increasingly greater affinities for the enzyme as described by Ondetti *et al.*[3] and Cushman *et al.*[70] in 1977. This program

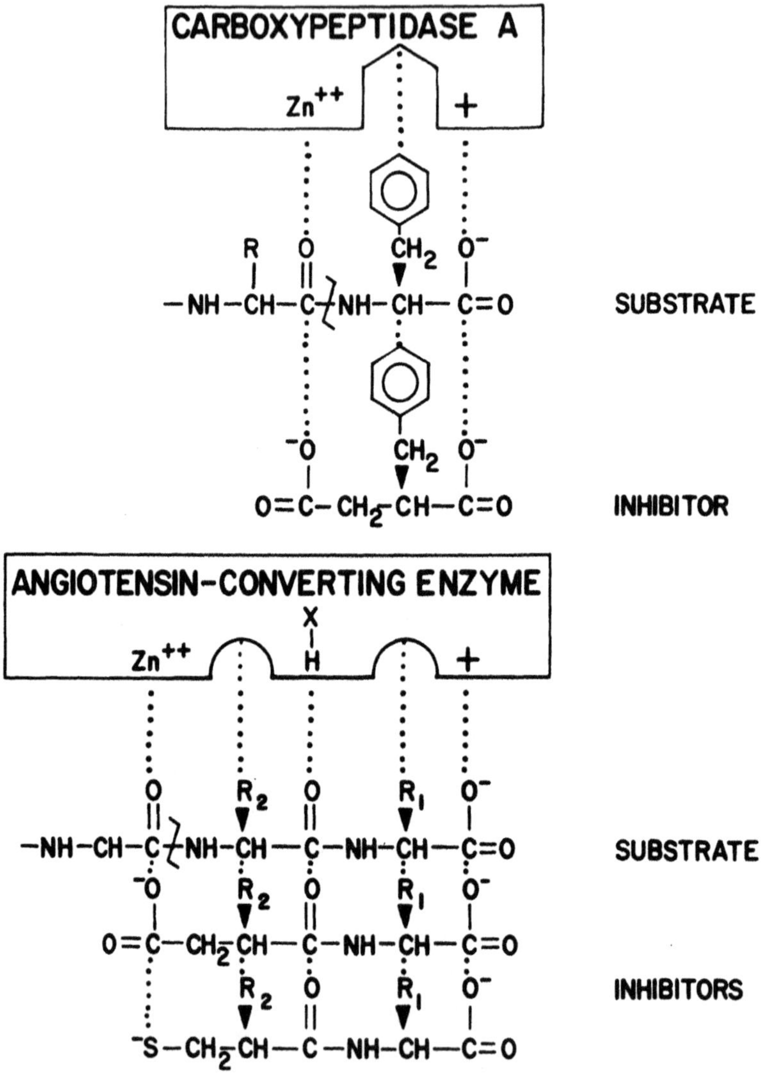

FIG. 2: Diagrammatic model of the active site of carboxypeptidase A and the analogous hypothetical active site of angiotensin-converting enzyme. For each enzyme, the known or proposed binding of peptide substrates and competitive inhibitors is indicated. *(Reprinted with permission from ref. 70).*

uncovered very high ACE inhibitory activity in a series of carboxyalkanoyl and mercaptoalkanoyl amino acids.

The hypothetical active site is based on the assumption that substrate binding and peptide bond cleavage by ACE occur in a manner similar to that of carboxypeptidase A (Fig. 2.).[3,22,70] Captopril (CAPOTEN®), which is D-3-mercapto-2-methylpropanoyl-L-proline (SQ 14,225), can be visualized as binding to ACE in the following manner. The negatively charged terminal carboxyl group interacts ionically with the same positively-charged residue of the enzyme that normally binds the terminal carboxyl of a peptide substrate; the amide carbonyl forms a hydrogen bond with a donor group on the enzyme; and the proline ring and methyl side-chains interact in a similar but unspecified manner as do the sidechains of the last two amino acid residues of a peptide substrate. The sulfhydryl group of captopril interacts strongly with the zinc ion of the enzyme. Captopril is one of the most potent members of this series of carboxyalkanoyl and mercaptoalkanoyl amino acids. Most importantly, captopril is active orally,[3,72,73] a feature highly desirable for chronic treatment of hypertension.

2C. <u>In vitro Inhibition of Converting Enzyme</u>

Teprotide and captopril are competitive inhibitors of purified ACE of rabbit lung with K_i values (enzyme-inhibitor dissociation constants) of 1.0×10^{-7} and 1.7×10^{-9}M, respectively.[21,23] On a molar basis, captopril is about 24 times more potent than teprotide as an inhibitor of rabbit lung ACE. The relative specificities of inhibitory activities by these compounds is apparent when each is tested against five other common peptidases (carboxypeptidase A, carboxypeptidase B, trypsin, chymotrypsin, and leucine aminopeptidase). Teprotide inhibits these peptidases only at concentrations about 600 to 3,000 times higher than that required to inhibit ACE. Captopril inhibits 4 of these peptidases (3 carboxypeptidases and 2 endopeptidases) at concentrations about 40,000 to 70,000 times higher than that needed to inhibit ACE. Captopril, however, inhibits leucine aminopeptidase at a concentration approximately 230 times greater than it's inhibitory IC_{50} *versus* rabbit lung ACE.[22]

When tested on excised guinea pig ileum, a specific inhibitor of ACE or kininase II should inhibit the contractile effect of AI (but not of AII) and augment the contractile effect of bradykinin.[59,71] On a weight and molar basis, respectively, captopril is ten and two times as potent as teprotide in inhibiting the effect of a single concentration of AI. Captopril, on a weight and molar basis, respectively, is about four times and four-fifths as potent as teprotide in augmenting the contractile effect of a single concentration of bradykinin. Under these particular conditions, Rubin *et al.*[72,73] found that the inhibitory IC_{50} (*versus* AI) and the augmenting AC_{50} (*versus* bradykinin) of captopril are about 5 and 1 ng/ml (0.023 and 0.0032 μM) respectively.

Further evidence for relatively high specificity of the activity of teprotide and captopril is also shown on excised smooth muscle. Amongst 11 agonists (other than AI or bradykinin) tested *in vitro* on a total of 5 types of vascular and non-vascular smooth muscle preparations, teprotide and captopril in concentrations 500 or 20,000 times higher than their respective IC_{50}'s versus AI, had little or no effect either on smooth muscle tone or on the contractile or relaxant action of each of the agonists.[22,59,72]

2D. In Vivo Inhibition of Converting Enzyme

The changes in both the aortic pressor responses to intravenous (i.v.) AI and AII and in the vasodepressor responses to i.v. BK and ACh were determined in conscious normotensive rats before and after dosage with captopril.[72,73] In related tests in conscious normotensive dogs, the systemic pressor response to i.v. AI and AII were determined; in most of these tests with captopril in dogs, heart rate, transthoracic EKG's, and peripheral venous plasma renin activity (PRA) were monitored.[73,74]

In fasted unanesthetized Sprague-Dawley normotensive rats (NR), single oral doses of 0.1-1.0 mg/kg of captopril produced, within the first 5-10 min, dose-related inhibition of the pressor response to AI; half-recovery times (t 1/2's) ranged from about 75 to 145 min. However, the pressor responses to AII or to l- norepinephrine, as well as resting mean blood pressure (MBP), were unaltered by these oral doses of captopril.[72,73]

Graded inhibition of the pressor effects of AI was obtained in conscious NR receiving single i.v. doses of 0.01-1.0 mg/kg of captopril, although t 1/2's were much shorter than after oral dosage, ranging from about 8 to 55 min.[72,73] The pressor responses to AII as well as resting MBP were again unchanged after this i.v. dose-range of captopril in conscious NR. Single oral doses of captopril were about one-eighth as effective as i.v. doses in terms of maximum inhibition, but the duration of inhibition of orally administered captopril was about 3-4 times longer than that achieved after i.v. captopril. The average p.o. and i.v. doses of captopril which reduced the pressor response to AI by 50% were about 0.17 and 0.02 mg/kg, respectively, in the NR. Little or no change in the reproducibility of captopril-induced inhibition of the pressor effect of AI occurred after short-term repeated i.v. or p.o. doses of captopril in NR.[72,73]

In unanesthetized NR, single oral doses of 0.01-1.0 mg/kg of captopril augmented and prolonged, at least twofold, the transient vasodepressor effect of BK, but not of ACh, particularly after the higher dose range. Resting MBP showed little or no change after the lower dose range. After 1.0 mg/kg of captopril, MBP showed a gradual average decrease of about 10%-20%, possibly related to the interaction with residual BK still circulating after the relatively large doses of BK.[72,73]

Intravenous doses of captopril, 0.31-1.0 mg/kg, inhibited the pressor response to AI, but not to norepinephrine, in conscious rabbits; the AII pressor response was slightly enhanced by the higher doses of captopril.[75] The vasopressor responses in rabbits and/or rats to i.v. serotonin, tyramine, or vasopressin, and the vasodepressor responses to i.v. isoproterenol, ACh, or prostaglandin E_2 were not affected by captopril, again demonstrating the relative specificity of captopril as an _in vivo_ inhibitor of ACE.[72,73,75-77] In conscious normotensive rabbits, inhibition of ACE with captopril, as judged by inhibition of the pressor responses to i.v. AI, markedly enhanced the magnitude and duration of the BK-induced hypotension.[76] Although in anephric rabbits the control hypotensive responses to i.v. BK were similar to those of normal rabbits,[75,76] the enhancement of BK's vasodepressor response by captopril in anephric rabbits was significantly smaller than that observed in normal rabbits.[76] Indomethacin, 2.5 mg/kg i.v., markedly attenuated the enhanced response to BK in normal rabbits, while in anephric rabbits, the attenuation was smaller than that observed in normal rabbits.[75,76] These results suggested to the authors[75,76] that, after inhibition of ACE in the rabbit, renal prostaglandins may have played a major role in the BK-induced hypotension, while any contribution of extrarenal prostaglandins may have been small. Since indomethacin did not interfere with ACE inhibition induced by captopril nor did indomethacin alter the pressor effect of AII and norepinephrine in these rabbits, the possibility of a mechanism other than inhibition of prostaglandin biosynthesis in explaining the observed effects appears to be unlikely.[75,76] Bilateral nephrectomy in rabbits did not interfere with the inhibitory effects of captopril on AI pressor responses.[76]

Unanesthetized normotensive dogs that had received single oral doses, 0.03-3.0 mg/kg, of captopril showed graded inhibition in degree and/or duration of the i.v. AI pressor responses.[74] About 85%-95% inhibition of the AI pressor response occurred within 15-30 min after 0.1-3.0 mg/kg p.o.; t 1/2's were generally longer than those seen in the rat after comparable doses. These oral doses of captopril in unanesthetized dogs produced little or no inhibition of the pressor response to AII and 3-10 fold increases in plasma renin activity.[74]

In anesthetized open-chest dogs, captopril caused a dose-dependent inhibition of the pressor as well as of the renal vasoconstrictor effects of AI.[78] The renal vasoconstrictor effects of AI were more susceptible (ID_{50} < 10 μg/kg i.v.) to inhibition by captopril than were the systemic pressor effects (ID_{50} = 37 μg/kg i.v.). Maximal inhibition of the pressor and vasoconstrictor effects of AI was seen after 100 μg/kg i.v. of captopril. Pressor responses to AII were not affected by captopril, whereas the renal vasoconstrictor effects of AII were enhanced.[78]

In chloralose-anesthetized cats, captopril antagonized the pressor responses to i.v. AI in a dose-related manner (maximum inhibition at about 310 μg/kg of captopril i.v.) but captopril did not alter the pressor responses to AII. Intravenous captopril had no effect on pressor responses to centrally administered AI or AII, whereas centrally administered captopril produced dose-related decreases to centrally administered AI but not AII. Thus, captopril does not appear to cross the blood-brain barrier to any significant degree but can inhibit central ACE if administered directly into the brain.[79]

In anesthetized rhesus monkeys, captopril had an ID_{50} of 6 μg/kg i.v. against AI pressor responses.[72]

In normotensive conscious humans, captopril produced dose-dependent reductions of i.v. AI pressor responses after oral administration of 1-20 mg of captopril.[80] Onset of action occurred within 15 min and declined to 40%-50% after 4 hr. The threshold inhibitory dose was about 1 mg, with a maximal effect occurring at 20 mg. Captopril, at 1-20 mg, had no effect on AII pressor responses in man.[80]

3. Effects on Blood Pressure

A. Normotensive Models

In salt-replete rats, cats, rabbits, and humans, intravenous or oral administration of captopril, or intravenous teprotide resulted in little (6-9%) or no decrease in blood pressure in doses up to 100 mg/kg[58,65,63,72,74,75,78,81-87] However, in salt-depleted rats, daily administration of captopril in the drinking water (0.5 mg/ml) resulted in blood pressure reductions greater than 30%.[86]

Unlike other species, sodium-replete dogs showed a significant dose-related reduction in blood pressure after either intravenous or oral administration of captopril, an effect directly related to the degree of AI inhibition.[74] In anesthetized dogs, captopril decreased blood pressure despite bilateral nephrectomy or inhibition of AII receptors by saralasin.[88]

In sodium-depleted animals or man, both captopril and teprotide caused substantial reductions in blood pressure as a consequence of the activation of the renin-angiotensin system caused by salt loss.[82,83,84,87,89]

B. Renal Hypertension

In 2-kidney, 1-clip renal hypertensive rats (2K-RHR), a model considered to be typical of renin-dependent hypertension in the first few weeks, captopril (1-30 mg/kg p.o.) caused dose-related reductions in mean arterial blood pressure (MBP) of up to 65 mm Hg when given daily for 2 days.[85]

In 2K-RHR with benign hypertension, captopril in the drinking water for 7 days reduced MBP from 133 $\pm$ 5 to 98 $\pm$ 3 mm Hg, whereas the same dosage regimen reduced MBP of 2K-RHR with malignant hypertension from 192 $\pm$ 5 to 108 $\pm$ 3 mm Hg within 24 hr.[90]

In chronic studies, captopril (30 mg/kg by gavage) reduced systolic blood pressure of conscious 2K-RHR, previously clipped unilaterally for 6 weeks. In addition, captopril maintained its antihypertensive action after daily oral administration for over 6 months[73,91] (Fig. 3). Only slight and inconsistent tolerance was noted in 2K-RHR, an effect attributed to a slowly developing sympathetic component since blood pressure could be normalized by additional treatment with guanethidine.[91] In all studies, captopril consistently produced a rapid reduction in systolic blood pressure, usually within 4 hr after the first dose. In contrast, return of blood pressure to predrug levels after cessation of captopril dosage required from 5 to 7 days. Although hydralazine caused an initially greater reduction in systolic blood pressure in 2K-RHR than captopril, rapid and virtually complete tolerance developed to its hypotensive effect within 4 weeks of daily oral dosing. The relative lack of tolerance to the effects of captopril may be related to a lack of sodium retention that normally occurs with other antihypertensive drugs[73,91].

Intermittent or chronic diuretic therapy had no effect on systolic blood pressure of 2K-RHR, results similar to those of other studies using either dietary sodium restriction or diuretics.[92-94] However, diuretic administration together with captopril, either intermittently or chronically, caused greater reductions in systolic blood pressure than either drug alone both in acute and chronic 2K-RHR (Fig. 3).

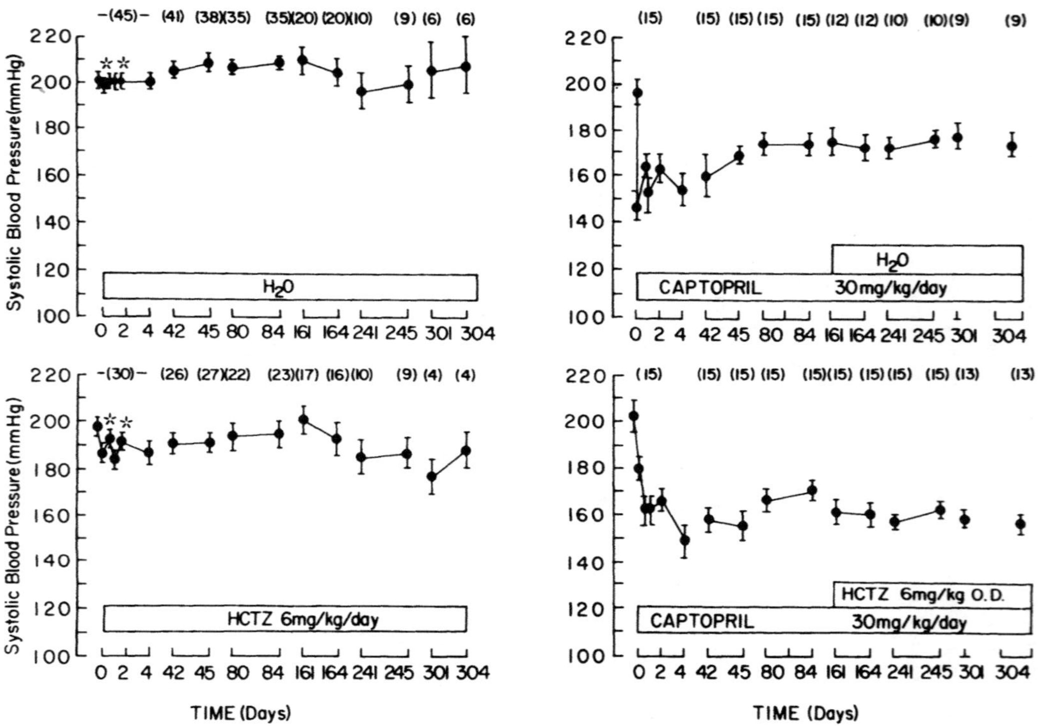

FIG. 3: Effects of daily oral treatment with water, hydrochlorothiazide (HCTZ), captopril, or captopril plus HCTZ on systolic blood pressure of two-kidney, one-clip renal hypertensive rats. Parentheses indicate number of animals per group. Values shown are mean ± S.E.M.

Daily treatment of 2K-RHR with captopril also resulted in a significant reduction in relative heart weights within 30 days of dosage, in comparison with vehicle-treated 2K-RHR which was maintained throughout the 6-month dosage period. The survival of 2K-RHR showed a dramatic increase in rats receiving captopril alone and an even further increase when captopril was combined with the diuretic hydrochlorothiazide in comparison with either water-treated controls or rats receiving the diuretic alone (Fig. 4). The increased survival is probably related to the antihypertensive effect since neither hydrochlorothiazide alone nor hydralazine chronically reduced systolic blood pressure or increased survival rate.[91,95]

Four weeks after surgery in a group of 14 2-kidney 2-wrapped hypertensive unanesthetized dogs, seven dogs were dosed orally each day for the next 9 weeks with captopril (31 mg/kg) and the other seven dogs were dosed with lactose placebo. The indirect mean blood pressures of the captopril-treated group were 25-50 mm Hg lower than those of the placebo-treated group. Blood pressures gradually returned to hypertensive levels similar to the placebo-treated group after captopril dosage was stopped during the next 4 weeks.[73]

Teprotide was also effective in reducing blood pressure in 2-kidney renal hypertensive rats[63,96-98], and in humans with renal hypertension.[66-68,99]

C. One Kidney, One-Clip Hypertension

In one-kidney, one-clip hypertensive rats (1K-RHR), hypertension is thought to be maintained by a nonrenin-dependent mechanism. In 1K-RHR with either benign or malignant hypertension, captopril was very effective in reducing MBP. However, in contrast with the renin-dependent 2K-RHR, marked reductions in MBP were not obtained until after several days of dosing with captopril.[73,86,100]

In 1K-RHR rats and dogs, oral administration of captopril before and after renal artery clipping delayed but did not prevent the onset of hypertension.[101,102]

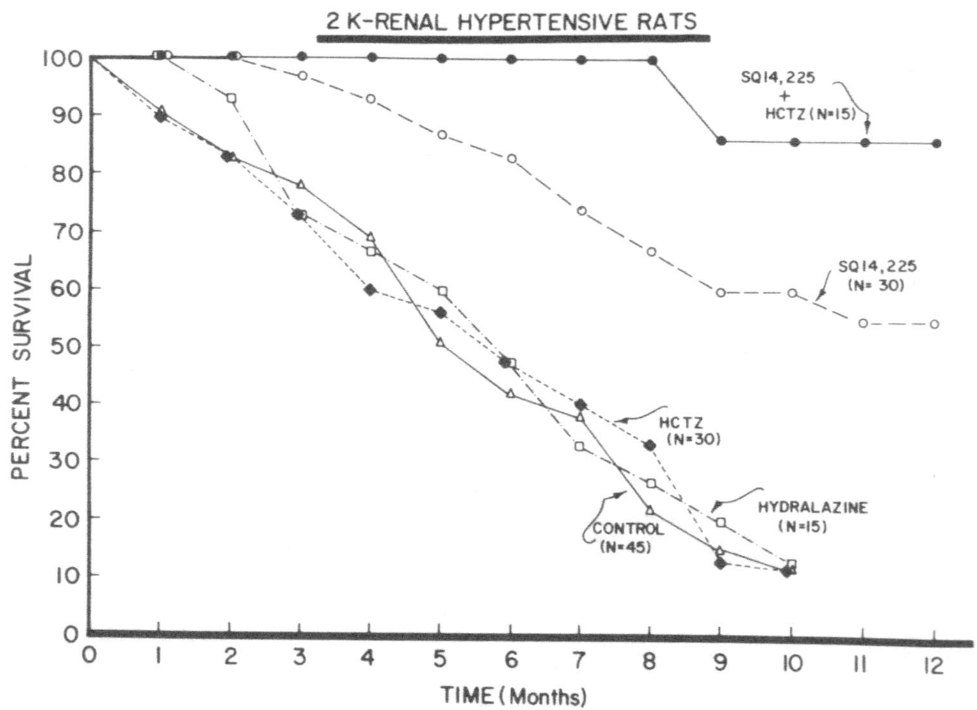

FIG. 4: Survival of two-kidney, one-clip renal hypertensive rats treated daily with either water (control), hydrochlorothiazide (HCTZ), hydralazine, captopril (SQ 14,225) or captopril + HCTZ. See Fig. 3 for details.

Teprotide was also found to be effective in reducing blood pressure of 1-kidney, 1-clip hypertensive dogs[83,103-105], rabbits[106] and mice[107].

D. Genetic (Spontaneous) Hypertension

In conscious, adult spontaneously hypertensive rats (SHR) of the Okamoto-Aoki strain, single oral doses of captopril ranging from 3 to 100 mg/kg caused maximum reductions in blood pressure of up to 25%.[73,85] Captopril was also effective in reducing blood pressure in stroke-prone SHR, the maximum reduction in blood pressure being greater than that observed in SHR.[73,108]

The effects of hydralazine (3 mg/kg) and captopril (100 mg/kg) on mean arterial blood pressure were examined in SHR after daily oral dosing for 2 weeks or 3 or 6 months. Captopril caused progressive, cumulative reductions in blood pressure resulting in normalization of pressure after 6 months of dosing (Fig. 5). No tolerance was observed. Hydralazine had less effect on blood pressure than captopril with no accumulation of effect being noted. Reductions in heart size paralleled the changes in blood pressure, with normalization of cardiac hypertrophy occurring after captopril but not hydralazine.[109]

In addition to reducing blood pressure in SHR with established hypertension, captopril (100 mg/kg in the drinking water) was able to completely prevent the development of hypertension in weanling SHR on drug for 16 weeks. Similar results were obtained in weanling SHR maintained on captopril for up to 12 weeks. Discontinuation of captopril after 4, 8 or 12 weeks resulted in the usual development of hypertension[110] (Fig. 6).

In the conscious New Zealand strain of genetic hypertensive rats, captopril, 30 mg/kg p.o. produced significant decreases in blood pressure.[73]

Teprotide has also been reported to reduce blood pressure in SHR when sufficiently high parenteral doses are used.[85]

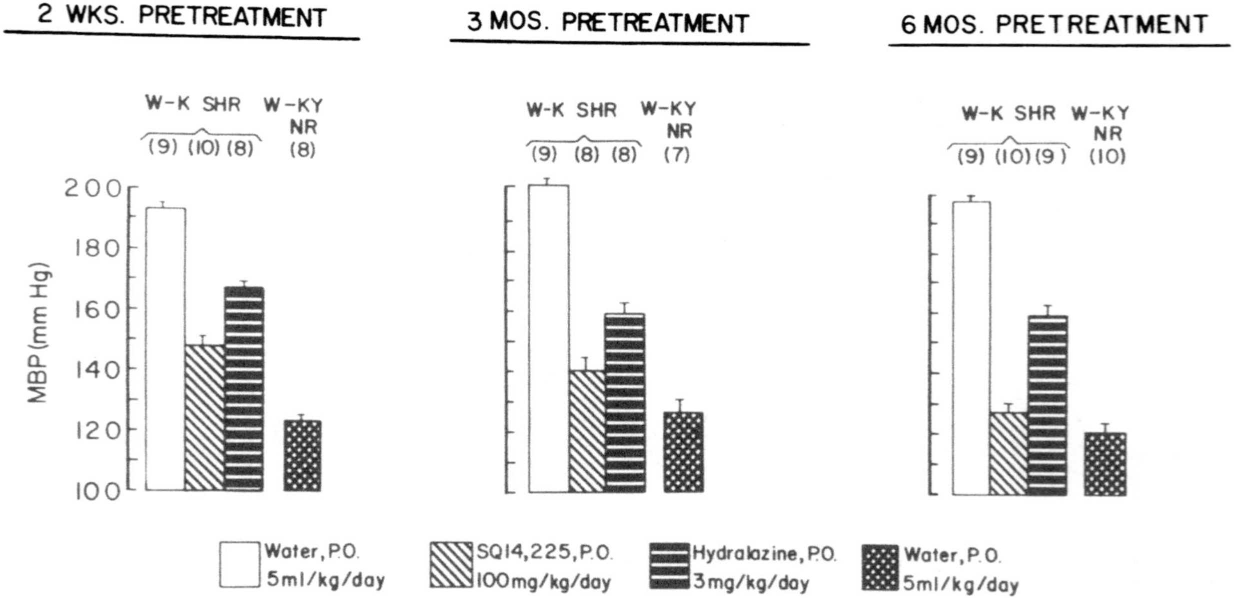

FIG. 5: Effects of daily oral dosing with water, captopril (SQ 14,225), or hydralazine on mean blood pressure (MBP) of spontaneously hypertensive rats after 2 weeks, 3 or 6 months of treatment. Also shown are the MBP's of normotensive WKY (W-KY NR) dosed with water. Parentheses indicate number of animals per group.

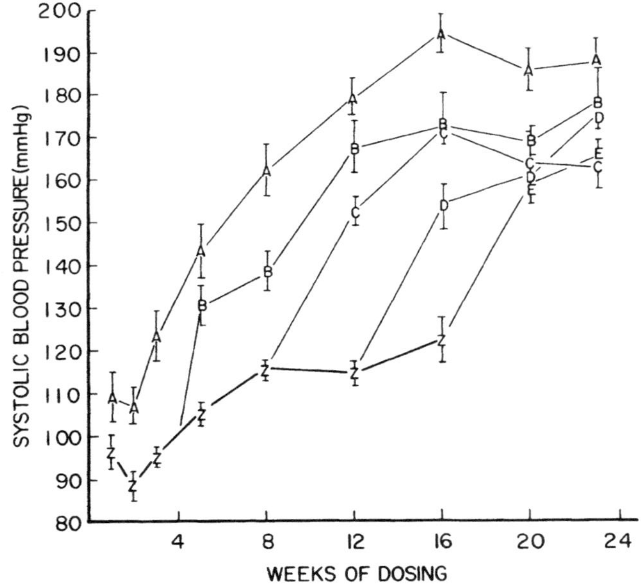

FIG. 6: Effect of captopril (100 mg/kg in drinking water) on systolic blood pressure of weanling (4 week old) SHR. Line A represents untreated controls and line Z represents SHR dosed with captopril. Lines B, C, D and E represent blood pressures of SHR after removal from captopril therapy. *(Reprinted with permission from ref. 110).*

E. DOCA-Salt Hypertension

Daily oral dosage with 10 to 100 mg/kg of captopril for 4 to 21 days had no consistent effect on blood pressure in DOCA-salt hypertensive rats.[73,111]

F. Other Models of Hypertension

In anesthetized hypertensive aortic-ligated rats (ligation between the two renal arteries), parenteral administration of captopril, 4 to 7 days post-ligation, produced moderate to marked decreases in diastolic blood pressure and slightly less decreases in systolic blood pressure.[85]

4. Antihypertensive Actions in Man

Captopril has been found to be active in most forms of human hypertension, with the exception of primary aldosteronism. Further reductions of blood pressure were obtained with either concomitant diuretic treatment or dietary sodium restriction.

Captopril, 25 to 1,000 mg/day administered to 19 hypertensive patients fed a 100 mEq sodium diet for 8 to 10 days, reduced arterial pressure by 28 mm Hg (-22.5%) in eight high-renin, and 22 mm Hg (-19.5%) in six normal-renin patients. In five low-renin patients, arterial pressure decreased 8.4%. Furthermore, the decrease in mean blood pressure was related to the pretreatment level of upright plasma renin activity.[112,113]

Case et al.[114] studied the effect of captopril in 19 hypertensive subjects, all of whom were either refractory or intolerant to conventional antihypertensive therapy. Six patients had renal artery stenosis and high-renin profiles and the other 12 had essential hypertension (two high-renin, nine medium-renin, and two low-renin). A total daily intake of 100 mEq of Na+ and 60 mEq of K+ was maintained in this series. Blood pressure fell at least 10% after captopril and the maximal allowed dose of 1,000 mg/day was reduced to 400 mg/day. In this study, an initial hypotensive response was observed followed by a later secondary reduction. There was a good correlation between the initial antihypertensive effect and a secondary decrease in blood pressure, especially in the subjects with pretreatment plasma renin activity levels greater than 2 ng AI/ml/hr. In eight high-renin patients, blood pressures on the 10th day were similar to those observed after 6 months of continuous treatment. Acceptable blood pressure control with captopril alone occurred in 14 of the 19 patients; four other patients, however, required the addition of a diuretic to achieve similar degrees of blood pressure control.

In a similar report by Atlas et al.[115] captopril was studied in 23 hypertensive patients for 10 days on a constant sodium and potassium diet. Fourteen of the patients were essential hypertensives (two high-renin, six normal-renin, and six low-renin), seven had renal hypertension (all high renin), and two were hypertensives with renal stenosis (normal-renin). After a period of 3 weeks without any medication, dose range studies of 2 or 3 days duration were performed; the maximum daily dose was 800 mg/day, the maintenance doses 150 to 800 mg/day, and average doses 325 to 450 mg/day. Blood pressure fell in response to the first dose of captopril in 22 of the 23 patients, then tended to revert transiently to control levels during the first few days of treatment and then fell again, reaching a nadir after 7 to 10 days of treatment.

Cody et al.[116] examined the hemodynamic effects of up to 1,000 mg/day of captopril for at least 3 days in eight hypertensive patients (four with essential and four with renovascular hypertension). Mean arterial pressure decreased by 22 mm Hg in this group. Two of the patients who did not respond initially showed a decrease in arterial pressure when sodium intake was reduced. Hemodynamic responses to head-up tilt were not affected by captopril regardless of sodium intake. Pulmonary hemodynamics showed little or no change and plasma volume increased slightly.

Brunner and associates[117] studied the antihypertensive effect of captopril in 22 hypertensive patients, 17 of whom were followed for periods of 1 to 7 months. Eight subjects had essential hypertension, eight renovascular hypertension, and six hypertension associated with chronic renal failure. Of these 22 patients, eight had high plasma renin activity according to the urinary sodium index, nine had normal activity, and five had low activity. Captopril decreased blood pressure significantly in all patients, including the low-renin group, with no evidence of tolerance or orthostatic hypotension (Fig. 7). The degree of blood pressure reduction was modestly correlated with the baseline plasma renin activity. Increasing the dose of captopril from 25 to 200 mg b.i.d. did not increase the degree of antihypertensive effect but did prolong its duration. In the course of the study, a ceiling dose of 400 mg/day was adopted. Four of the patients required additional diuretic therapy, three of whom had associated renal failure.

In seven patients with hypertension of renal failure, most of whom were refractory to multiple antihypertensive drug therapy, captopril (200 mg b.i.d. for 4-6 days for at least 4 weeks) reduced blood pressure by 23 mm Hg. Five of these patients needed additional treatment with a diuretic to reduce blood pressure further.[118,119]

In another six patients (four with essential hypertension and two with renovascular hypertension), captopril at 25 to 100 mg doses produced a significant decrease in blood pressure in patients who did not respond or responded only poorly to an infusion of saralasin.[120]

Bravo and Tarazi (121) administered captopril for at least 3 days at oral doses of 80 to 1,000 mg/day to 10 essential hypertensives and to seven patients with renovascular hypertension. These patients had

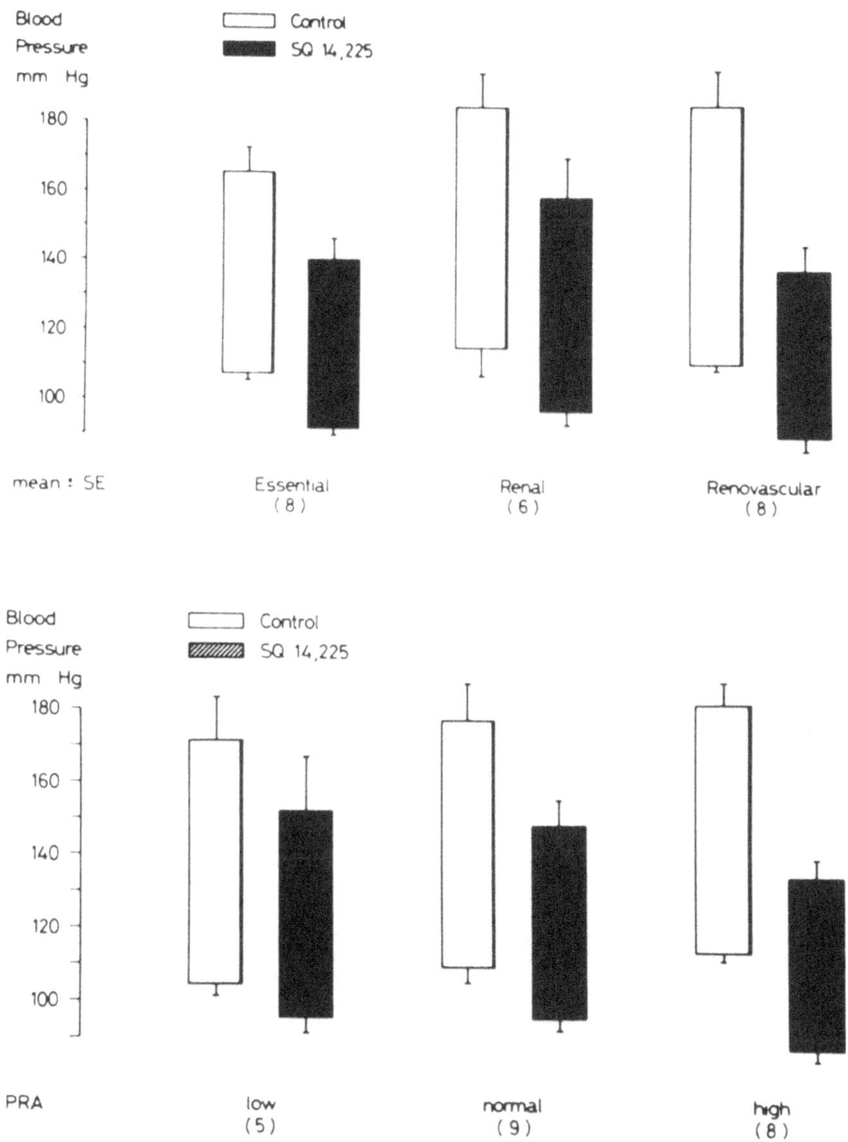

FIG. 7: Effects of captopril (SQ 14,225) on systolic and diastolic blood pressure of hypertensive patients according to etiology (top panel) and plasma renin activity (bottom panel). *(Reprinted with permission from ref. 117).*

previously been designated as having drug-resistant hypertension, diuretics, sympatholytics, and peripheral vasodilating agents having been used with only minimal effect, excessive side effects, and/or lack of compliance. In eight of the subjects blood pressure was reduced to the normotensive range when maintained on normal dietary sodium during therapy with captopril; the degree of reduction was not predictable by plasma renin activity. Another seven patients with residual hypertension showed further decreases in blood pressure when dietary sodium was reduced to 10 mEq/day. No rebound hypertension occurred when treatment with captopril was temporarily stopped. Orthostatic hypotension did not occur during captopril therapy.

Gavras _et al._[122] investigated the antihypertensive effect of captopril, 400 to 1,000 mg for 3 to 24 weeks, in 12 hypertensive patients (six had essential hypertension with three low, two normal, and one high renin, and six had renovascular hypertension with three normal, and three high renin levels). Four of these patients had been refractory to other antihypertensive medication. Blood pressure decreased in all patients from 177/110 to 136/88 mm Hg; heart rate increased 5 beats/min.

Eleven patients with essential hypertension and four patients with renovascular hypertension maintained on a daily intake of 100 mEq of sodium and 60 mEq of potassium received captopril, 10 to 1,000 mg/day for periods ranging from 3 days to 12 months.[123] Normalization of blood pressure occurred in all but three patients, one with severe renovascular hypertension whose pressure decreased 11%, one with severe essential hypertension whose pressure fell 27%, and one with essential hypertension whose pressure decreased 8.5%. Diastolic pressures of the 15 patients fell an average of 24%. The average control diastolic pressure in the essential hypertensives was 115 mm Hg and fell to 90 mm Hg; average diastolic pressure in renovascular hypertensives decreased from 111 mm Hg to 94 mm Hg.

Another 15 patients (four renovascular and 11 essential hypertensives) received captopril (200-600 mg/day) for periods ranging up to 6 months. Blood pressures were normalized by 1 week in nine subjects on a regular salt diet, five of whom were essential hypertensives. Mean blood pressure decreased 23 mm Hg. Most of the other six patients showed some reduction in pressure after addition of a diuretic; however, the poorest response was obtained in two of these subjects who were found to have primary aldosteronism.[124]

In 16 patients who were poorly responsive or intolerant prior to antihypertensive therapy, captopril (75-600 mg/day) caused significant decreases in diastolic blood pressure in 15 patients, who were maintained on therapy for 3 to 6 months.[125]

5. Hemodynamics

A. Animal Studies

In all species tested thus far, captopril reduced total peripheral resistance while either having no effect on, or increasing cardiac output.[78,126,127]

In anesthetized normotensive dogs, captopril (0.31 mg/kg i.v.) decreased systolic, diastolic, and mean blood pressure as well as total and renal vascular resistance.[78] Heart rate was only transiently and slightly increased, whereas cardiac output, left ventricular dp/dt, mean pulmonary pressure, and pulmonary vascular resistance were unchanged. Despite the decrease in blood pressure, renal blood flow increased significantly after captopril.[78] In another acute study, captopril decreased renal arterial pressure and increased renal blood flow, whereas inulin clearance remained constant.[128]

Similarly, in conscious SHR, captopril decreased total peripheral resistance with either no change or an increase in cardiac output.[126,127]

Captopril increased blood flow to all organs examined in SHR, the changes being significant in heart, kidney, and splanchnic organs.[126]

In salt-depleted normotensive dogs, captopril decreased arterial pressure, increased renal blood flow and decreased glomerular filtration rate.[89]

B. Human Studies

In human hypertensives on 100 mM of sodium/day, a reduction in mean arterial pressure from 149 $\pm$ 5 to 127 $\pm$ 8 mm Hg after 3 to 7 days of captopril (320 to 1,000 mg/day) was due totally to a reduction in total peripheral resistance with no significant change in cardiac index, pulmonary wedge pressure, heart rate, pulmonary artery pressure, or vascular resistance; plasma volume was slightly but significantly increased. Similar results were found in hypertensives on a 10 mM sodium/day diet.[116]

Virtually identical hemodynamic changes after captopril were reported by others.[123]

6. Endocrinological Effects

A. Renin Activity

In normotensive rats, rabbits, and dogs as well as in renal hypertensive rats and dogs, SHR, and in hypertensive man,[73,74,85,88,95,109,114] captopril, and teprotide (see 14,129) caused 2- to 15-fold increases in plasma renin activity (PRA). These increases in PRA are thought to be mainly a result of inhibition of negative feed-back mechanisms by AII on the juxtaglomerular apparatus. Reductions of circulating AII caused by ACE inhibition with captopril should result in increased renal secretion of renin in an attempt by the body to restore reduced AII levels. In hypertensive models, reduction of blood pressure by captopril might also contribute to the elevated plasma renin activity through a compensatory reflex increase in sympathetic nerve activity to the kidney. Interestingly, β-blockade with propranolol prevented the increase in PRA caused by captopril in SHR just as β-blockade inhibited the rise in PRA caused by saralasin in man.[130-132] This suggests that the final stimulus to increased PRA in situations of reduced AII activity is activation of sympathetic pathways.

B. Angiotensin I, Angiotensin II, Aldosterone, and Bradykinin

By inhibiting the conversion of AI to AII, captopril caused an increase in circulating AI and a decrease in AII levels in both animals and humans.[124,133-135] As a consequence of the reductions of AII formation, aldosterone secretion is also inhibited by captopril. Captopril has been shown to reduce aldosterone levels in human hypertension, whether it be essential, renovascular, or chronic renal failure hypertension.[114,115,117,121,122,125] Remarkably consistent reductions in plasma aldosterone levels ranging from 47 to 62% have been demonstrated by many investigators with urinary aldosterone levels showing parallel reductions of 42 to 65%. Similarly, plasma aldosterone concentrations were reduced in both 1- and 2-kidney, 1-clip malignant hypertensive rats as well as in normotensive salt-depleted dogs and rats.[86,89,90]

No changes in aldosterone secretion have been observed after captopril in normotensive salt-replete rats or 1-kidney, 1-clip benign hypertensive rats.[86,90] Similarly, urinary aldosterone levels showed no change in SHR treated daily for 6 months with captopril in which blood pressure had been reduced to normal levels.[73,109]

In contrast to the consistent changes observed in the renin-angiotensin-aldosterone system after captopril, reports of changes in the kallikrein-kinin system have been variable. In human essential hypertensive patients, no changes in kallikrein excretion were reported,[136] whereas McCaa[89] showed a marked reduction in urinary kallikrein excretion after captopril in sodium-depleted normotensive dogs. Plasma bradykinin levels have been shown to be elevated in human normotensive patients whose blood pressure was unaltered by captopril,[137] as well as in sodium-depleted normotensive dogs whose blood pressure was markedly decreased by captopril.[89] However, other investigators have reported either no change or a moderate decrease in plasma bradykinin levels in human hypertensive patients after captopril.[134,135]

7. Water, Sodium, and Potassium

In some studies, captopril has been shown to increase sodium and water excretion without affecting potassium excretion. Thus, in sodium-depleted normotensive rats and dogs, 1- and 2K-RHR, urinary water and sodium excretion were increased by captopril.[86,89] In sodium-replete normotensive rats and in young as well as mature SHR, captopril either did not affect or increased water and sodium excretion.[77,86,109,127,138] In anesthetized normotensive dogs, captopril did not change urinary sodium or potassium excretion probably because of the reductions in renal perfusion pressure, since maintenance of this pressure resulted in significant natriuresis and kaliuresis by captopril.[128]

The effects of captopril in human hypertension on sodium and water excretion were variable, investigators having reported increases, decreases, or no change.[114,115,117] Potassium excretion and plasma levels remained unaltered in most cases, although slight increases have also been reported.[115,122,123]

8. Congestive Heart Failure

The renin-angiotensin-aldosterone system plays a critical role in the sodium retention, edema, and ascites observed in animal models of congestive heart failure, whether the failure is associated with low- or high-cardiac output. Infusions of the AII antagonist saralasin[139] or the peptide ACE inhibitor teprotide[140] decreased arterial pressure and aldosterone secretion in dogs with thoracic inferior vena cava constriction, and also prevented the formation of peripheral edema and ascites in this model of low-output congestive failure.

Captopril has also been found to be very effective in a caval constriction model of low-output failure in dogs.[141] Captopril caused similar changes in dogs with high-output failure caused by an aortic-cava fistula.[142]

In human patients with chronic heart failure refractory to therapy with digitalis glycosides and diuretics, relatively small doses of captopril (25-150 mg) caused a decrease in arterial blood pressure, heart rate, pulmonary wedge pressure, and systemic vascular resistance while increasing cardiac index. The effects were generally maximal 1½ hr after captopril administration. Although PRAs were elevated in these patients, the effects of captopril did not correlate with pre-drug PRA. Favorable hemodynamic changes were maintained in chronic heart failure patients on long-term therapy with captopril.[143-150]

9. Hemorrhagic Shock

In cats in hemorrhagic shock, infusion of captopril resulted in a significantly higher final arterial pressure than those given saline, significant reductions in circulating lysosomal hydrolase, total plasma proteolysis, and myocardial depressant factor. The beneficial hemodynamic patterns observed after captopril in these animals were apparently all due to ACE inhibition, although the relative contributions of AII synthesis inhibition and BK potentiation were not known.[151]

10. Mechanism of Action

There is no evidence to suggest that captopril exerts the majority of its pharmacological effects through any other mechanism except inhibition of ACE. It is not a vasodilator, has no direct effects on sympathetic or parasympathetic nerve function, does not interfere with receptor activation of any agonist tested nor does it enter the brain.

In renovascular hypertension where high plasma renin activity is apparent, reductions in blood pressure by inhibition of ACE with captopril is rapid, and consistent with the onset of inhibition of pressor responses to AI. Furthermore, antagonists of AII receptors such as saralasin[152] are also effective in reducing blood pressure in renovascular hypertensive with high PRA.

The effectiveness of captopril in hypertension associated with low or normal PRA is, however, not so readily understood. Thus, while it is tempting to suggest that captopril acts to reduce blood pressure in chronic renal hypertension by the same mechanism as in acute renal hypertension - that is, blockade of renin-angiotensin system through ACE inhibition - several observations appear to militate against this explanation. As opposed to acute 2K-RHR, PRA values are not elevated in chronic 2K-RHR[153,154] nor are renal vein PRA's of the contralateral unclipped kidney.[155] As opposed to marked reductions of blood pressure in acute 2K-RHR, chronic 2K-RHR show no change in blood pressure to infusions of AII antagonists.[93,153] Finally, bilateral nephrectomy does not importantly reduce blood pressure of chronic 2K-RHR whereas this procedure is very effective in acute 2K-RHR.[155] Therefore, it seems inescapable that increased plasma renin activity is not responsible for maintaining the hypertensive state of chronic 2K-RHR.

Similar problems exist in trying to explain the effectiveness of captopril, both in preventing hypertension in weanling SHR[110] and normalizing it in established hypertension of adult SHR.[109] PRA values of adult SHR are either no different or lower than normotensive adult rat models.[109,156] Thus, it seems paradoxical that captopril should be able to normalize the

the blood pressure of SHR simply by inhibiting the renin-angiotensin system, especially since administration of AII receptor antagonists or AII antibodies[153,157] have no effect on the blood pressure of SHR. Miyazaki and Yamamoto[158] recently demonstrated that a synthetic phosphatidylethanolamine inhibitor of renin was capable of reducing blood pressure of both renal hypertensive rats and SHR. Thus, the possibility must be considered that plasma renin activity *per se* is also not a good determinant of the significance of the renin-angiotensin system in maintaining blood pressure of SHR, a suggestion also postulated by Horovitz.[159]

Similarly, the effectiveness of captopril in 1K-RHR, another model of normal renin hypertension, has also been amply demonstrated[73,86] with no good clues to its mode of action.

Several possible mechanisms of the antihypertensive activity still related to ACE inhibition may account for the effectiveness of captopril in low or normal renin states of hypertension:

A. Arterial Wall Renin - Arterial vascular tissue of several species including man contains all of the components necessary for the local generation of AII.[160,161] This local vascular AII formation is of functional significance, responds to typical stimuli, and is elevated in chronic 2K-RHR as well as adult SHR (no reports are available for 1K-RHR) in which PRA's are normal.[161,162] Thus, inhibition of locally generated AII might explain how renin inhibitors and captopril reduce blood pressure in these models.[63] AII antagonists may not be effective because of their relatively large molecular bulk which does not allow them to penetrate to the local vascular site of AII formation. Support for such a hypothesis is provided by studies in 2K-RHR and SHR in which acute bilateral nephrectomy either raised or had no effect on blood pressure[164-166], whereas ACE inhibition by teprotide (SQ 20,881) still caused reductions in the acutely nephrectomized (formerly 2K-RHR) hypertensive rats.[166]

B. Bradykinin Accumulation - ACE is the same enzyme as kininase II which is responsible for the inactivation of bradykinin, inhibition of which causes marked potentiation of the cardiovascular effects of bradykinin (BK). Thus, it is conceivable that accumulation of BK might occur with chronic inhibition of ACE and be particularly responsible for some of its effects. This is a very difficult hypothesis to test since local accumulation of BK might not be reflected in circulating plasma or urine levels but which could have very profound cardiovascular effects through renal vasodilation, diuresis, natriuresis, and inhibition of sympathetic function. Unfortunately, the literature is not consistent in relation to BK levels after captopril, some investigators reporting increases in kinin levels[89,137] while others report either no change[134] or a decrease.[135]

Indirect evidence against the involvement of kinins in the cardiovascular effects of captopril comes from several sources: a) as shown in Table 1, pretreatment of SHR with the kallikrein inhibitor aprotonin (60,000 KIU twice daily for 3 days) did not prevent captopril's antihypertensive effect, suggesting that de novo synthesis of kinins is not involved in the observed action of captopril in this model.

On the other hand, an intact renin-angiotensin system appears to be essential for the actions of captopril. Inhibition of renin with the renin inhibitor URI-73A (25 mg/kg i.m. daily for 3 days) [100] in SHR resulted in a modest reduction in MBP of about 33 mm Hg. Concomitant therapy with captopril in these SHR did not add to the effect observed after the renin inhibitor by itself.[166a] b) Captopril has been demonstrated to be without effect either in the development, or in the established state, of DOCA-salt hypertension.[73,111] Since this model has been demonstrated to have a a high kallikrein activity[167], one would anticipate that captopril might be

Table 1

Effect of Kallikrein Inhibition with Aprotonin (Trasylol®) on the Antihypertensive Action of Captopril in SHR

Treatment Group	Control Mean Blood Pressure (MBP, mm Hg)	MBP After Aprotonin[a]	MBP After Treatment[b]
Captopril 30 mg/kg p.o. (n = 6)	181.7 ± 5.7	148.3 ± 6.1*	118.5 ± 4.3
Water 5 ml/kg p.o. (n=6)	183.5 ± 5.8	150.7 ± 10.3*	146.2 ± 7.0

[a]60,000 KIU/rat twice daily for 4 days; MBP is 6 hrs after the last dose of aprotonin and immediately prior to treatment with captopril.

[b]Maximum change observed over a 4-hr period of observation.

*p <0.01 *vs*. control

**p <0.01 *vs*. aprotonin treated MBP

quite effective in reducing blood pressure through inhibition of kinin degradation. 3) The hemodynamic consequences of BK administration - namely, vasodilation with marked reflex increases in heart rate and cardiac output - are in contrast to the actual changes associated with captopril and d) the reduction in blood pressure after captopril requires several days to return to control levels after discontinuation of drug. Since converting enzyme activity returns to control levels well before blood pressure does[127,168] and since BK has a very short half-life,[169] significant BK accumulation seems unlikely as an obvious mechanism of antihypertensive action. It is also important to note that increases in plasma BK levels have been observed in normotensive patients whose blood pressures were unchanged after captopril. Moreover, no changes in BK levels have been observed in groups of hypertensive patients in whom blood pressure was dramatically reduced by captopril.

C. Prostaglandin Release - Enhanced cardiovascular responsiveness to BK administration has been shown in one study to be partially mediated through the release of renal prostaglandins.[76] However, neither the antihypertensive nor the renal vasodilating properties of captopril are apparently due to prostaglandins since indomethacin has no effect on these parameters when given before captopril in SHR.[130] Furthermore, captopril did not change urinary PGE_2 levels in renovascular hypertensive human patients.[116]

D. Kidneys and Adrenal Glands - Captopril has been consistently shown to decrease aldosterone secretion in hypertensive animals[90] and humans.[114,122] Since this is undoubtedly a consequence related to inhibition of AII formation, it is difficult to determine how much of the antihypertensive action of captopril is directly related to reductions in AII formation compared to how much is due to reductions in aldosterone secretion. Certainly, the acute antihypertensive effects of captopril in SHR are not due to aldosterone inhibition since reductions in blood pressure were unaltered after bilateral adrenalectomy, either prior to or following captopril administration.[166a] On the other hand, the reductions of blood pressure in sodium-depleted normotensive dogs after chronic captopril could be reversed by simultaneous administration of aldosterone sufficient to raise plasma levels to normal.[90] It seems likely that the chronic effects - perhaps the secondary reduction in pressure observed in human patients - of captopril in hypertensive patients involves inhibition of aldosterone release.

It is apparent that the kidneys are necessary for the antihypertensive action of captopril in conditions of salt-repletion. Sham bilateral nephrectomy was without effect on the antihypertensive action of captopril in both SHR and chronic (16-week) 2K-RHR. However, actual bilateral nephrectomy after captopril administration resulted in the return of blood pressure to pre-drug levels despite a second dose of captopril following nephrectomy in both SHR and 2K-RHR.[166a]

E. <u>Sodium and Water Excretion</u> - Captopril has been shown to cause increases in sodium and water excretion and therefore might decrease blood pressure by reducing sodium content and/or flux in vessels, as well as by reducing plasma volume. However, this appears unlikely since the diuretic and natriuretic actions of captopril can be dissociated from changes in blood pressure. In both animal [86,109,127] and human hypertension[115,116] captopril can reduce blood pressure with associated increases, decreases or unaltered excretion of sodium. Also, captopril does not reduce plasma volume.[100,116,123]

In conclusion, captopril is an effective antihypertensive agent in most forms of hypertension. Its only method of action appears to be inhibition of ACE but the consequences of this inhibition are complicated and not clarified as yet. Degrees of blood pressure reduction are poorly correlated with pre-drug PRA but greater reductions in blood pressure are observed in high renin hypertensive states.

Acknowledgments

The authors gratefully acknowledge the efforts of Mrs. Helen Stofko and Mrs. Carol Materniak in typing the manuscript.

REFERENCES

1. Ondetti, M.A., Williams, N.J., Sabo, E.F., Pluščec, J., Weaver, E.R., and Kocy, O., Angiotensin-converting enzyme inhibitors from the venom of Bothrops jararaca. Isolation, elucidation of structure, and synthesis, Biochemistry, 10, 4033, 1971.

2. Cheung, H.S. and Cushman, D.W., Inhibition of homogeneous angiotensin-converting enzyme of rabbit lung by synthetic venom peptides of Bothrops jararaca, Biochem. Biophys. Acta, 293, 451, 1973.

3. Ondetti, M.A., Rubin, B., and Cushman, D.W., Design of specific inhibitors of angiotensin-converting enzyme: new class of orally active antihypertensive agents, Science, 196, 441, 1977.

4. Laragh, J.H. and Sealey, J.E., The renin-angiotensin-aldosterone hormonal system and regulation of sodium, potassium and blood pressure homeostasis, in Handbook of Physiology, Sect. 8, Renal Physiology, Orloff, J. and Berliner, R.W., Eds., Amer. Physiol. Soc., Washington, D.C., 1973, 815.

5. Davis, J.O. and Freeman, R.H., Mechanisms regulating renin release, Physiol. Rev., 56, 1, 1976.

6. Ganten, D. and Gross, F., Interference with the renin-angiotensin system and their effects on high blood pressure, in Handbook of Experimental Pharmacology, Vol. 39, Antihypertensive Agents, Gross, F., Ed., Springer-Verlag, Berlin, 1977, chap. 11.

7. Peach, M.J., Renin-angiotensin system: biochemistry and mechanisms of action, Physiol. Rev., 57,313, 1977.

8. Vecsei, P., Hackenthal, E., and Ganten, D., The renin-angiotensin-aldosterone system, Klin. Wochenschr., 56 (Suppl. 1), 5, 1978.

9. Pisano, J.J. and Austen, K.F., Eds., Chemistry and biology of the kallikrein-kinin system in health and disease, U.S. Govt. Printing Office, Washington, D.C., DHEW Publication No. (NIH) 76-791, 1974, chap. 1-76.

10. Vane, J.R. and McGiff, J.C., Possible contributions of prostaglandins to the control of blood pressure, Circ. Res., 36/37, I-68, 1975.

11. Carretero, O.A. and Scicli, A.G., The renal kallikrein-kinin system in human and in experimental hypertension, Klin. Wochenschr., 56 (Suppl. 1), 113, 1978.

12. Dusting, G.J., Moncada, S., and Vane, J.R., Prostaglandins, their intermediates and precursors: cardiovascular actions and regulatory roles in normal and abnormal circulatory systems, Progr. Cardiovasc. Dis., 21, 405, 1979.

13. Nasjletti, A. and Malik, K.U., Relationships between the kallikrein-kinin and prostaglandin systems, Life Sci., 25, 99, 1979.

14. Cushman, D.W. and Ondetti, M.A., Inhibitors of angiotensin-converting enzyme, Progr. Med. Chem., 17, in press, 1980.

15. Erdös, E.G., Angiotensin I converting enzyme, Circ. Res., 36, 247, 1975.

16. Erdös, E.G., Commentary. The kinins, Biochem. Pharmacol., 25, 1563, 1976.

17. Erdös, E.G., Conversion of angiotensin I to angiotensin II, Am. J. Med., 60, 749, 1976.

18. Erdös, E.G., Ed., Handbook of Experimental Pharmacology, Vol. 25, Bradykinin, kallidin, and kallikrein, Springer-Verlag, Berlin, 1970, chap. 1-9.

19. Erdös, E.G., Ed., Handbook of Experimental Pharmacology, Vol. 25 Suppl., Bradykinin, kallidin, and kallikrein, Springer-Verlag, Berlin, 1979, chap. 1-17.

20. Page, I.H. and Bumpus, F.M., Eds., Handbook of Experimental Pharmacology, Vol. 37, Angiotensin, Springer-Verlag, Berlin, 1974, p. 1-519.

21. Ondetti, M.A. and Cushman, D.W., Inhibitors of the renin-angiotensin system, Annu. Rep. Med. Chem., 13, 82, 1978.

22. Cushman, D.W., Cheung, H.S., Sabo, E.F., Rubin, B., and Ondetti, M.A., Development of specific inhibitors of angiotensin I converting enzyme (kininase II), Fed. Proc., 38, 2778, 1979

23. Levinsky, N.G., The renal kallikrein-kinin system, Circ. Res., 44, 441, 1979.

24. McGiff, J.C. and Wong, P.Y-K, Compartmentalization of prostaglandins and prostacyclin within the kidney: implications for renal function, Fed. Proc., 38, 89, 1979.

25. Tigerstedt, R. and Bergman, P.G., Niere und Kreislauf, Skand. Arch. Physiol., 8, 223, 1898.

26. Goldblatt, H., Lynch, J., Hanzal, R.F., and Summerville, W.W., Studies on experimental hypertension. Production of persistent elevation of systolic blood pressure by means of renal ischemia, J. Exp. Med., 59, 347, 1934.

27. Braun-Menéndez, E.J., Fasciolo, J.C., Leloir, L.F., and Muñoz, J.M., La substancia hipertensora de la sangre del riñon isquemiado, Rev. Soc. Arg. Biol., 15, 420, 1939.

28. Page, I.H. and Helmer, O.M., A crystalline pressor substance (angiotonin) resulting from the reaction between renin and renin activator, J. Exp. Med., 71, 29, 1940.

29. Braun-Menéndez, E.J. and Page, I.H., Suggested revision of nomenclature-angiotensin, Science, 127, 242, 1958.

30. Skeggs, L.T., Marsh, W.H., Kahn, J.R., and Shumway, N.P., The existence of two forms of hypertensin, J. Exp. Med., 99, 275, 1954.

31. Lentz, K.E., Skeggs, L.T., Woods, K.R., Kahn, J.R., and Shumway, N.P., The amino acid composition of hypertensin II and its biochemical relationship to hypertension, J. Exp. Med., 104, 183, 1956.

32. Elliott, D.F. and Peart, W.S., The amino acid sequence in a hypertensin, Biochem J., 65, 246, 1957.

33. Skeggs, L.T., Lentz, K.E., Kehr, J.R., Shumway, N.P., and Woods, K.R., Amino acid sequence of hypertensin II, J. Exp. Med., 104, 193, 1956.

34. Schwyzer, R., Iselin, B., Kappeler, H., Rinker, B., Rittel, W., and Zuber, H., Syntheses von Hypertensin-peptiden, Chimie (Aarau), 11, 335, 1957.

35. Bumpus, F.M., Schwarz, H., and Page, I.H., Synthesis and pharmacology of the octapeptide angiotensin, Science, 125, 886, 1957.

36. Carpenter, C.C.J., Davis, J.O., and Ayers, C.R., Relation of renin, angiotensin II and experimental renal hypertension to aldosterone secretion, J. Clin. Invest., 40, 2026, 1961.

37. Genest, J., Biron, P., Koiw, E., Nowaczynski, W., Chretein, M., and Boucher R., Adrenocortical hormones in human hypertension and their relation to angiotensin, Circ. Res., 9, 775, 1961.

38. Gross, F., Renin und hypertensin, physiologische oder pathologische wirkstoffe? Klin. Wochenschr., 36, 693, 1958.

39. Laragh, J.H., The role of aldosterone in man: evidence for regulation of electrolyte balance and arterial pressure by renal-adrenal system which may be involved in malignant hypertension, J. Am. Med. Assoc., 174, 293, 1960.

40. Mulrow, P.J., Ganong, W.F., Cera, G., and Kuljian, A., Nature of aldosterone stimulating factors in dog kidneys, J. Clin. Invest., 41, 505, 1962.

41. Ng, K.K.F. and Vane, J.R., Conversion of angiotensin I to angiotensin II, Nature, 216, 762, 1967.

42. Blair-West, J.R., Coghlan, J.P., Denton, D.A., Funder, J.W., Scoggins, B.A. and Wright, R.D., The effect of the heptapeptide (2-8) and the hexapeptide (3-8) fragments of angiotensin II on aldosterone secretion, J. Clin. Endocrinol. Metab., 32, 575, 1971.

43. Goodfriend, T.L. and Peach, M.J., Angiotensin III; (des-aspartic acid^1)-angiotensin II. Evidence and speculation for its role as an important agonist in the renin-angiotensin system. Circ. Res., 36/37, I-38, 1975.

44. McCaa, R.E., Aldosterone response to long term infusion of angiotensin II and angiotensin III in conscious dogs before and after dietary sodium restriction, Endocrinology, 103, 458, 1978.

45. Werle, E., Discovery of the most important kallikreins and kallikrein inhibitors, in Handbook of Experimental Pharmacology, Vol. 25, Bradykinin, Kallidin and Kallikrein, Erdös, E.G., Ed., Springer-Verlag, Berlin, 1970, chap. 1.

46. Eisen, V. and Vogt, W., Plasma kininogenases and their activators, in Handbook of Experimental Pharmacology, Vol. 25, Bradykinin, Kallidin and Kallikrein, Erdös, E.G., Ed., Springer-Verlag, Berlin, 1970, chap. 3.

47. Webster, M.E., Kallikreins in glandular tissues; recommendations for nomenclature and units, in Handbook of Experimental Pharmacology, Vol. 25, Bradykinin, Kallidin and Kallikrein, Erdös, E.G., Ed., Springer-Verlag, Berlin, 1970, p. 131 and p. 659.

48. Rocha e Silva, M., Beraldo, W.T., and Rosenfeld, G., Bradykinin, a hypotensive and smooth muscle stimulating factor released from plasma globulin by snake venoms and by trypsin, Am. J. Physiol., 156, 261, 1949.

49. Elliott, D.F., Horton, E.W., and Lewis, G.P., Actions of pure bradykinin, J. Physiol., 153, 473, 1960.

50. Boissonnas, R.A., Guttman, S., and Jaquenod, P.A., Synthese de la L-arginyl-L-prolyl-L-prolyl-glycyl-L-phénylalanyl-L-seryl-L-prolyl-L-phénylalanyl-L-arginine, un nonapeptide présentant les propriétés de la bradykinine, Helv. chem. Acta, 43, 1349, 1960.

51. Igic, R., Erdos, E.G., Yeh, H.S.J., Sorelic, K., and Nakajima, T., Angiotensin I converting enzyme of the lung, Circ. Res., 30/31, II-51, 1972.

52. Ferreira, S.H., A bradykinin-potentiating factor (BPF) present in the venom of Bothrops jararaca, Brit. J. Pharmacol., 24, 163, 1965.

53. Bakhle, Y.S., Conversion of angiotensin I to angiotensin II by cell-free extracts of dog lung, Nature, 220, 919, 1968.

54. Ferreira, S.H., Bartelt, D.C., and Greene, L.J., Isolation of bradykinin potentiating peptides from Bothrops jararaca venom, Biochemistry, 9, 2583, 1970.

55. Ferreira, S.H., Greene, L.J., Alabaster, V.A., Bakhle, Y.S., and Vane, J.R., Activity of various fractions of bradykinin potentiating factor against angiotensin-converting enzyme, Nature, 225, 379, 1970.

56. Stewart, J.M., Ferreira, S.H., and Greene, L.J., Bradykinin potentiating peptide PCA-Lys-Trp-Ala-Pro. An inhibitor of the pulmonary inactivation of bradykinin and conversion of angiotensin I to II, Biochem. Pharmacol., 20, 1557, 1971.

57. Cushman, D.W. and Cheung, H.S., Spectrophotometric assay and properties of the angiotensin-converting enzyme of rabbit lung, Biochem. Pharmacol., 20, 1637, 1971.

58. Engel, S.L., Schaeffer, T.R., Gold, B.I., and Rubin, B., Inhibition of pressor effects of angiotensin I and augmentation of depressor effects of bradykinin by synthetic peptides, Proc. Soc. Exp. Biol. Med., 140, 240, 1972.

59. O'Keefe, E.H., Kotler, D.G., Waugh, M.H., and Rubin, B., Inhibition and augmentation by peptide SQ 20,881 of contractile effects of angiotensin I (AI) and of bradykinin (B), respectively, on excised smooth muscle, Fed. Proc., 31, 511, 1972.

60. Kato, H. and Suzuki, T., Bradykinin-potentiating peptides from the venom of Agkistrodon halys blomhoffii. Isolation of five bradykinin potentiators and the amino acid sequence of two of them, potentiators B and C, Biochemistry, 10, 972, 1971.

61. Bakhle, Y.S., Inhibition of converting enzyme by venom peptides, in Hypertension, Genest, J. and Koiw, E., Eds., Springer-Verlag, Berlin, 1972, p. 541.

62. Greene, L.J., Camargo, A.C.M., Krieger, E.M., Stewart, J.M., and Ferreira, S.H., Inhibition of the conversion of angiotensin I to II and potentiation of bradykinin by small peptides present in Bothrops jararaca venom, Circ. Res., 30/31, II-62, 1972.

63. Engel, S.L., Schaeffer, T.R., Waugh, M.H., and Rubin, B., Effects of the nonapeptide SQ 20,881 on blood pressure of rats with experimental hypertension, Proc. Soc. Exp. Biol. Med., 143, 483, 1973.

64. Muirhead, E.E., Brooks, B., and Arora, K.K., Prevention of malignant hypertension by the synthetic peptide SQ 20,881, Lab. Invest., 30, 129, 1974.

65. Collier, J.G., Robison, B.F., and Vane, J.R., Reduction of pressor effects of angiotensin I in man by synthetic nonapeptide which inhibits converting enzyme, Lancet, 1, 72, 1973.

66. Gavras, H., Brunner, H.R., Laragh, J.H., and Vukovich, R.A., An angiotensin converting enzyme inhibitor to identify and treat vasoconstrictor and volume factors in hypertensive patients, N.Engl. J. Med., 291, 817, 1974.

67. Johnson, J.G., Black, W.D., Vukovich, R.A., Hatch, F.E., Jr., Friedman, B.I., Blackwell, C.F., Shenouda, A., Share, L., Shade, R.E., Acchiardo, S.R., and Muirhead, E.E., Treatment of patients with severe hypertension by inhibition of angiotensin-converting enzyme, Clin. Sci. Mol. Med., 48, 53s, 1975.

68. Case, D.B., Wallace, J.M., Keim, H.J., Weber, M.A., Sealey, J.E., and Laragh, J.H., Possible role of renin in hypertension as suggested by renin-sodium profiling and inhibition of converting enzyme, N. Engl. J. Med., 206, 641, 1977.

69. Krieger, E.M., Salgado, H.C., Assan, C.J., Greene, L.J., and Ferreira, S.H., Potential screening test for detection of overactivity of the renin-angiotensin system, Lancet, 1, 269, 1971.

70. Cushman, D.W., Cheung, H.S., Sabo, E.F., and Ondetti, M.A., Design of potent competitive inhibitors of angiotensin-converting enzyme. Carboxyalkanoyl and mercaptoalkanoyl amino acids, Biochemistry, 16, 5484, 1977.

71. Rubin, B., O'Keefe, E.H., Kotler, D.G., DeMaio, D.A., and Cushman, D.W., Use of excised guinea pig ileum as a predictive test for inhibitors in vivo of angiotensin-converting enzyme (ACE), Fed. Proc., 34, 770, 1975.

72. Rubin, B., Laffan, R.J., Kotler, D.G., O'Keefe, E.H., DeMaio, D.A., and Goldberg, M.E., SQ 14,225 (D-3-mercapto-2-methylpropanoyl-L-proline), a novel orally active inhibitor of angiotensin-converting enzyme, J. Pharmacol. Exp. Ther. 204, 271, 1978.

73. Rubin, B., Antonaccio, M.J., and Horovitz, Z.P., Captopril (SQ 14,225) (D-3-mercapto-2-methylpropanoyl-L-proline): a novel orally active inhibitor of angiotensin-converting enzyme and antihypertensive agent, Progr. Cardiovasc. Dis., 21, 183, 1978.

74. Harris, D.N., Heran, C.L., Goldenberg, H.J., High, J.P., Laffan, R.J., Rubin, B., Antonaccio, M.J., and Goldberg, M.E., Effects of SQ 14,225, an orally active inhibitor of angiotensin-converting enzyme on blood pressure, heart rate and plasma renin activity of conscious normotensive dogs, Eur. J. Pharmacol., 51, 345, 1978.

75. Murthy, V.S., Waldron, T.L., Goldberg, M.E., and Vollmer, R.R., Inhibition of angiotensin converting enzyme by SQ 14,225 in conscious rabbits, Eur. J. Pharmacol 46, 207, 1977.

76. Murthy, V.S., Waldron, T.L., and Goldberg, M.E., The mechanism of bradykinin potentiation after inhibition of angiotensin-converting enzyme by SQ 14,225 in conscious rabbits, Circu. Res., 43, I-40, 1978.

77. Rubin, B., Duchin, K.L., and Antonaccio, M.J., Effects of chronic captopril (C) on renal function and vascular reactivity in conscious Wistar-Kyoto (WKY) rats, Fed. Proc., 38, 851, 1979.

78. Murthy, V.S., Waldron, T.L., and Goldberg, M.E., Inhibition of angiotensin converting enzyme by SQ 14,225 in anesthetized dogs: hemodynamic and renal vascular effects, Proc. Soc. Exp. Biol. Med., 157, 121, 1978.

79. Vollmer, R.R. and Boccagno, J.A., Central cardiovascular effects of SQ 14,225, an angiotensin-converting enzyme inhibitor in chloralose-anesthetized cats, Eur. J. Pharmacol., 45, 117, 1977.

80. Ferguson, R.K., Brunner, H.R., Turini, G.A., Gavras, H., and McKinstry, D.N., A specific orally active inhibitor of angiotensin-converting enzyme in man, Lancet, 1, 775, 1977.

81. Bing, J. and Poulsen, K., Time course of changes in plasma renin after blockade of the renin system, Acta Path. Microbiol. Scand., Sect. A, 83, 454, 1975.

82. Haber, E., Sancho, J., Re, R., Burton, J., and Barger, A.C., The role of the renin-angiotensin-aldosterone system in cardiovascular homeostasis in normal man, Clin. Sci. Mol. Med., 48, 495, 1975.

83. Samuels, A.I., Miller, Jr.,E.D., Fray, J.C.S., Haber, E., and Barger, A.C., Renin-angiotensin antagonists and the regulation of blood pressure, Fed. Proc., 35, 2512, 1976.

84. Thurston, H. and Laragh, J.H., Prior receptor occupancy as a determinant of the pressor activity of infused angiotensin II in the rat, Circ. Res., 36, 113, 1975.

85. Laffan, R.J., Goldberg, M.E., High, J.P., Schaeffer, T. R., Waugh, M.H., and Rubin, B., Antihypertensive activity in rats of SQ 14,225, an orally active inhibitor of angiotensin converting enzyme, J. Pharmacol. Exp. Ther., 204, 281, 1978.

86. Bengis, R.G., Coleman, T.G., Young, D.B., and McCaa, R.E., Long-term blockade of angiotensin formation in various normotensive and hypertensive rat models using converting enzyme inhibitor (SQ 14,225), Circ. Res., 43 (Suppl. I), 45, 1978.

87. Jaeger, P., Ferguson, R. K., Brunner, H.R., Kirchertz, R., and Gavras, H., Mechanism of blood pressure reduction by teprotide (SQ 20,881) in rats, Kidney Int., 13, 289, 1978.

88. Vollmer, R.R., Boccagno, J.A., Harris, D.N., and Murthy, V.S., Hypotension induced by inhibition of angiotensin-converting enzyme in pentobarbital-anesthetized dogs, Eur. J. Pharmacol., 51, 39, 1978.

89. McCaa, R.E., Hall, J.E., and McCaa, C.S., The effects of angiotensin I-converting enzyme inhibitors on arterial blood pressure and urinary sodium excretion. Role of the renin-angiotensin and kallikrein-kinin systems, Circ. Res., 43 (Suppl. I), 32, 1978.

90. McCaa, R.E., McCaa, C.S., Bengis, R.G., and Guyton, A.C., Role of aldosterone in experimental hypertension, J. Endocrinol., 81, 69P, 1979.

91. Antonaccio, M.J., Rubin, B., Horovitz, Z.P., Mackaness, G., and Panasevich, R., Long-term efficacy of captopril (SQ 14,225) in 2-kidney renal hypertensive rats. Clin. Exp. Hypertension, 1, 505, 1979.

92. Brown, T.C., Davis, J.O., Olichney, M.J., and Johnston, C.I., Relation of plasma renin to sodium balance and arterial pressure in experimental renal hypertension, Circ. Res., 18, 475, 1966.

93. Gavras, H., Oliver, J.A., and Cannon, P.J., Interrelations of renin, angiotensin II, and sodium in hypertension and renal failure, Annu. Rev. Med., 27, 485, 1976.

94. Miksche, L.W., Miksche, U., and Gross, F., Effect of sodium restriction on renal hypertension and on renin activity in the rat, Circ. Res., 27, 973, 1970.

95. Rubin, B., Antonaccio, M.J., Goldberg, M.E., Harris, D.N., Itkin, I.G., Horovitz, Z.P., Panasevich, R.E., and Laffan, R.J., Chronic antihypertensive effects of captopril (SQ 14,225), an orally active angiotensin I-converting enzyme inhibitor in conscious 2-kidney renal hypertensive rats, Eur. J. Pharmacol., 51, 377, 1978.

96. Douglas, J.R., Jr., Johnson, E.M., Jr., Heist, J.F., Marshall, G.R., and Needleman, P., Is the peripheral sympathoadrenal nervous system necessary for renal hypertension?, J. Pharmacol. Exp. Ther., 196, 35, 1976.

97. Thurston, H. and Swales, J.D., Blood pressure response of nephrectomized hypertensive rats to converting enzyme inhibition: Evidence for persistent vascular renin activity, Clin. Sci. Mol. Med., 52, 299, 1977.

98. Riegger, A.J.G., Lever, A.F., Millar, J.A., Morton, J.J., and Slack, B., Correction of renal hypertension in rat by long term infusion of angiotensin inhibitors, Lancet, 2, 1317, 1977.

99. Gavras, H., Brunner, H.R., Laragh, J.H., Gavras, I., and Vukovich, R. A., The use of angiotensin converting enzyme inhibitor in the diagnosis and treatment of hypertension, Clin. Sci. Mol. Med., 48, 57S, 1975.

100. Sen, S., Smeby, R. R., Bumpus, F.M., and Turcotte, R.G., Role of renin-angiotensin system in chronic renal hypertensive rats, Hypertension, 1, 427, 1979.

101. Freeman, R.H., Davis, J.O., Watkins, B.E., Stephens, G.A., and DeForrest, J.M., Effects of continuous converting enzyme blockade on renovascular hypertension in the rat, Am. J. Physiol., 236, F21, 1979.

102. Watkins, B.E., Davis, J.O., Freeman, R.H., Stephens, G.A., and DeForrest, J.M. Effects of oral converting enzyme inhibitor (SQ 14,225) on one-kidney hypertension in the dog, Proc. Soc. Exp. Biol. Med., 157, 245, 1978.

103. Watkins, B.E., Davis, J.O., Freeman, R.H., DeForrest, J.M., and Stephens, G.A., Continuous angiotensin II blockade throughout the acute phase of one-kidney hypertension in the dog, Circ. Res., 42, 813, 1978.

104. Miller, E.D., Jr., Samuals, A.I., Haber, E., and Barger, A.C., Inhibition of angiotensin conversion in experimental renovascular hypertension, Science, 177, 1108, 1972.

105. Ayers, C.R., Vaughan, E.D., Jr., Yancey, M.R., Bing, K.T., Johnson, C.C., and Morton, C., Effect of 1-sarcosine-8-alanine angiotensin II and converting enzyme inhibitor on renin release in dog acute renovascular hypertension, Circ. Res., 34, I27, 1974.

106. Muirhead, E.E., Brooks, B., and Arora, K.K., Prevention of malignant hypertension by the synthetic peptide SQ 20,881, Lab. Invest., 30, 129, 1974.

107. Svendsen, U.G., Effects of the nonapeptide (SQ 20,881) on the blood pressure of conscious normotensive and chronic hypertensive mice, Acta Path. Microbiol. Scand., Sect. A, 85, 942, 1977.

108. Watanabe, T.X. and Sokabe, H., Acute vasodepressor effect of D-3-mercapto-2-methyl-propanoyl-L-proline (SQ 14,225) in the stroke-prone substrain of spontaneously hypertensive rats (SHRSP), Jap. J. Pharmacol., 29, 133, 1979.

109. Antonaccio, M.J., Rubin, B., Horovitz, Z.P., Laffan, R.J., Goldberg, M.E., Harris, D.N., and Zaidi, I. Effects of chronic treatment with captopril (SQ 14,225), an orally active inhibitor of angiotensin I-converting enzyme, in spontaneously hypertensive rats, Jap. J. Pharmacol., 29, 285, 1979.

110. Ferrone, R.A. and Antonaccio, M.J., Prevention of the development of spontaneous hypertension in rats by captopril (SQ 14,225), Eur. J. Pharmacol., In press.

111. Douglas, B.H., Langford, H.C., and McCaa, R.E., Response of mineralocorticoid hypertensive animals to an angiotensin I converting enzyme inhibitor, Proc. Soc. Exp. Biol. Med., 161, 86, 1979.

112. Atlas, S.A., Case, D.B., Sealey, J.E., McKinstry, D.N., and Laragh, J.H., Blunted aldosterone secretion, natriuresis and potassium retention during chronic aldosterone blockade in hypertensive patients, Clin. Res., 26, 361A, 1978.

113. Atlas, S.A., Case, D.B. Sealey, J.E., Sullivan, P.M., and Laragh, J.H., Involvement of the renin-angiotensin-aldosterone axis in the antihypertensive action of captopril (SQ 14,225), Circulation, 57/78 (Suppl. II), II-143, 1978.

114. Case, D.B., Atlas, S.A., Laragh, J.H., Sealey, J.E., Sullivan, P.A., and McKinistry,D.N., Clinical experience with blockade of the renin-angiotensin-aldosterone system by an oral converting-enzyme inhibitor (SQ 14,225, captopril) in hypertensive patients, Prog. Cardiovasc. Dis., 21, 195, 1978.

115. Atlas, S.A., Case, D.B., Sealey, J.E., Laragh, J.H., and McKinstry, D.N., Interruption of the renin-angiotensin system in hypertensive patients by captopril induces sustained reduction in aldosterone secretion, potassium retention and natriuresis, Hypertension, 1, 274, 1979.

116. Cody, R.J.,Jr., Tarazi, R.C., Bravo, E.L., and Fouad, F.M., Hemodynamics of orally-active converting enzyme inhibitor (SQ 14,225) in hypertensive patients. Clin. Sci. Mol. Med., 55, 453, 1978.

117. Brunner, H. R., Gavras, H., Waeber, B., Kershaw, G.R., Turini, G.A., Vukovich, R.A., and McKinstry, D.N., Oral angiotensin-converting enzyme inhibitor in long-term treatment of hypertensive patients, Ann. Intern. Med., 90, 19, 1979.

118. Brunner, H.R., Gavras, H., Turini, G.A., Waeber, B., and Wauters, J.P., Long-term angiotensin blockade in hypertensive patients with chronic renal failure Clin. Res., 26, 459A, 1978.

119. Brunner, H.R., Waeber, B., Wauters, J.P., Turini, G., McKinstry, D., and Gavras, H., Inappropriate renin secretion unmasked by captopril (SQ 14,225) in hypertension of chronic renal failure, Lancet, 2, 704, 1978.

120. Baker, K.M. Vaughn, E.D., Jr., Johns, D.W., Ayers, C.R., and Carey, R.M., Antihypertensive effects of angiotensin blockade: SQ 14,225 versus P113, Clin. Res., 26, 779A, 1978.

121. Bravo, E. L. and Tarazi, R.C., Converting enzyme inhibition with an orally active compound in hypertensive man, Hypertension, 1, 39, 1979.

122. Gavras, H., Brunner, H.R., Turini, G.A., Kershaw, G.R., Tifft, C.P., Cuttelod, S., Gavras, I., Vukovich, R.A., and McKinstry, D.N., Antihypertensive effect of the oral angiotensin converting enzyme inhibitor SQ 14,225 in man, N. Engl. J. Med., 298, 991, 1978.

123. Sullivan, J.M., Ginsburg, B.A., Ratts, T.E., Johnson, J.G., Barton, B.A., Kraus, D.H., McKinstry, D.N., and Muirhead, E.E., Hemodynamic and antihypertensive effects of captopril, an orally active angiotensin converting enzyme inhibitor, Hypertension, 1, 397, 1979.

124. Favre, L., Frazer, M., McKinstry, D.N., and Hollifield, J.W., Chronic antihypertensive therapy with an oral converting-enzyme inhibitor (CEI), Circulation, 57/58 (Suppl. II), I-57, 1978.

125. McKinstry, D.N., Willard, D.A., and Vukovich, R.A., Antihypertensive and hormonal effects of the converting enzyme inhibitor, captopril, alone or combined with hydrochlorothiazide, Clin. Pharmacol. Ther., 25, 237, 1979.

126. Ferrone, R.A. and Heran, C.L., Hemodynamic effects of SQ 14,225 and guanethidine in spontaneously hypertensive rats. Circulation, 57/58 (Suppl. II), II-144, 1978.

127. Muirhead, E. E., Prewitt, R. L., Jr., Brooks, B., and Brosius, W. L., Jr., Antihypertensive action of the orally active converting enzyme inhibitor (SQ 14,225) in spontaneously hypertensive rats, Circ. Res. (Suppl. I), 43: 153, 1978.

128. Duchin, K. L. and Steinbacher, T.E., Effects of captopril (SQ 14,225) on renal function in the dog. Kidney Int., 14, 693, 1978.

129. Ondetti, M.A. and Cushman, D.W., Angiotensin-Converting Enzyme Inhibitors, in The Biochemical Regulation of Blood Pressure, Soffer, R.L., Ed., John Wiley and Sons, New York, In press.

130. Antonaccio, M.J., Harris, D., Goldenberg, H., High, J.P., and Rubin, B., The effects of captopril, propranolol, and indomethacin on blood pressure and plasma renin activity in spontaneously hypertensive and normotensive rats, Proc. Soc. Exp. Biol. Med., In press.

131. Brunner, H.R., Gavras, H., and Laragh, J.H., Hypertension in man. Exposure of the renin and sodium components using angiotensin II blockade. Circ Res. 34/35 (Suppl. I), 135, 1974.

132. Pettinger, W.A. and Mitchell, H.C., Renin release, saralasin, and the vasodilator-beta blocker drug interaction in man, N. Engl. J. Med., 292, 1214, 1975.

133. Atkinson, A.B., Brown, J.J., Lever, A.F., Morton, J.J., Frazer, R., and Robertson, J.I.S., Changes in plasma angiotensin II during captopril therapy in renal hypertension and intractable essential hypertension. Proceedings of the 6th Scientific Meeting of the International Society on Hypertension, Goteborg, June 11-13, p. 121, 1979.

134. Matthews, G., McGrath, B., and Johnston, C., Hormonal changes with long-term converting enzyme inhibition by captopril in essential hypertension, Proceedings of the 6th Scientific Meeting of the International Society on Hypertension, Goteborg, June 11-13, p. 156, 1979.

135. Millar, J.A., and Johnston, C.I., The effect of captopril (SQ 14,225) on circulating levels and clearance of angiotensin I and bradykinin in man, dog, and rabbit, Proceedings of the 6th Scientific Meeting of the International Society on Hypertension, Goteborg, June 11-13, p. 157, 1979.

136. Keim, H.J., Bindel, G., Distler, A., Fleckenstein, P., and Cordes, U., Long-term treatment of essential hypertension (EH) with the oral converting enzyme inhibitor SQ 14,225, Proceedings of the 6th Scientific Meeting of the International Society on Hypertension, Goteborg, June 11-13, p. 144, 1979.

137. McKinstry, D.N., Singhvi, S.M., Kripalani, K.J., Dreyfuss, J., Willard, D.A., and Vukovich, R.A., Disposition and cardiovascular-endocrine effects of an orally active angiotensin-converting enzyme inhibitor, SQ 14,225, in normal subjects, Clin. Pharmacol. Ther., 23, 121, 1978.

138. Crofton, J.T., Share, L., and Horovitz, Z.P., The effect of SQ 14,225 on systolic blood pressure and urinary excretion of vasopressin in the developing SH rat. Hypertension, 1, 462, 1979.

139. Johnson, J.A. and Davis, J.O., Effects of a specific competitive antagonist of angiotensin II on arterial pressure and adrenal steroid secretion in the dog, Circ. Res., 32 (Suppl. I), I159, 1973.

140. Watkins, L.J., Burton, J.A., Huber, E., Cant, T.R., Smith, F.W., and Barger, A.C., The renin-angiotensin system in congestive failure in conscious dogs, J. Clin. Invest., 57, 1606, 1976.

141. Freeman, R.H., Davis, J.O., Williams, G.M., DeForrest, J.M., Seymour, A.A., and Rowe, B.P., Effects of the oral converting enzyme inhibitor, SQ 14,225, in a model of low cardiac output in dogs, Circ. Res., 45, 540, 1979.

142. Williams, G.M., David, J.O., Freeman, R.H., DeForrest, J.M., Seymour, A.A., and Rowe, B.P. Effects of the oral converting enzyme inhibitor, SQ 14,225, in experimental high output failure, Am. J. Physiol., 236, F541, 1979.

143. Adler, R., Chatterjee, K., Ports, T., Hiramatsu, B., and Parmley, W., Beneficial hemodynamic effects of angiotensin converting enzyme inhibitor in chronic refractory heart failure, Am. J. Cardiol., 43, 404, 1979.

144. Davis, R., Ribner, H.S., Keung, E., Sonnenblick, E.H., and LeJemtel, T.H., Treatment of chronic congestive heart failure with captopril, an oral inhibitor of angiotensin-converting enzyme, N. Engl. J. Med., 301, 117, 1979.

145. Turini, G.A., Gribic, M., Brunner, H.R., Waeber, B., and Gavras, H., Improvement of chronic congestive heart failure by oral captopril, Lancet, 1, 1213, 1979.

146. Mason, D.T., Awan, N.A., Hermanovich, J. and Joye, J.A., Oral captopril in congestive heart failure: efficacy by cardiac catherization, forearm plethysmography, nuclear scintigraphy, echography, treadmill exercise symptoms, Circulation, 59/60 (Suppl. II), 230, 1979.

147. Levine, T.B., Carlyle, P.F., Gross, K.A., Franciosa, J.A. and Cohn, J.A., Hemodynamic and clinical response to captopril in congestive heart failure, Circulation, 59/60 (Suppl. II), 39, 1979.

148. Halperin, J.L., Creager, M.A., Faxon, D.P., Gavras, H. and Ryan, T.J., Chronic oral angiotensin inhibition for the treatment of refractory heart failure, Circulation, 59/60 (Suppl. II), 39, 1979.

149. Fouad, F.M., Cerino, J.M., Tarazi, R.C. and Bravo, E.L., Converting enzyme inhibition (CEI) in normotensive heart failure (HF): long term hemodynamic and humoral effects, Circulation, 59/60 (Suppl. II), 130, 1979.

150. Fouad, F.M., Cerino, J.M., Tarazi, R.C. and Bravo, E.L., Oral converting enzyme inhibitor in resistant heart failure, Clin. Res., 27, 673A, 1979.

151. Trache, G.J. and Lefer, A.M., Beneficial action of a new angiotensin-converting enzyme inhibitor (SQ 14,225) in hemorrhagic shock in cats, Circ. Res., 43, 576, 1978.

152. Hollenberg, N.K., Williams, G.H., Adams, D.F., Moore, T., Brown, C., Borucki, L.J Leung, F., Booli, S., Solomon, H.S., Passau, D. and Dluhy, R., Pharmacological interruption of the renin-angiotensin system, Medicine, 58, 115, 1979.

153. Carretero, O.A. and Gulati, O.P., Effects of angiotensin antagonist in rats with acute, subacute, and chronic two-kidney renal hypertension, J. Lab. Clin. Med., 91, 264, 1978.

154. Koletsky, S., Rivera-Velez, J.M., Marsh, D.G., and Pritchard, W.H., Relation of renal arterial pressure to activity of renin-angiotensin system in renal hypertension, Proc. Soc. Exp. Biol. Med., 125, 96, 1967.

155. Koletsky, S. and Rivera-Velez, J.M., Factors determining the success or failure of nephrectomy in experimental renal hypertension, J. Lab. Clin. Med., 76, 54, 1970.

156. Shiono, K. and Sokabe, H., Renin-angiotensin system in spontaneously hypertensive rats, Am. J. Physiol., 231, 1295, 1976.

157. Pals, D.T., Masucci, F.D., Denning, G.S., Jr., Sipos, F., and Fessler, D.C., Role of the pressor action of angiotensin II in experimental hypertension, Circ. Res., 29, 673, 1971.

158. Miyazaki, M. and Yamamoto, K., Synthetic phosphatidyl-ethanolamines as renin inhibitors, Proc. Soc. Exp. Biol. Med., 155, 468, 1977.

159. Horovitz, Z.P., Pharmacology and mechanism of action of inhibitors of the angiotensin converting enzyme in Pharmacology and Clinical Use of Angiotensin I Converting Enzyme Inhibitors, Drug Development and Evaluation, vol. 4, Gross, F. and Liedtke, R.K., Eds., Gustav Fischer Verlag, Stuttgart, 1980, p. 9-14.

160. Ganten, D., Hutchinson, J.S., Schelling, P., Ganten, U., and Fischer, H., The iso-renin angiotensin systems in extrarenal tissue, Clin. Exp. Pharmacol. Physiol., 3, 103, 1976.

161. Swales, J.D., Arterial wall or plasma renin in hypertension, Clin. Sci., 56, 293, 1979.

162. Sen, S., Smeby, R. R., and Bumpus, F.M., Renin in rats with spontaneous hypertension, Circ. Res., 31, 876, 1972.

163. Asaad, M.M. and Antonaccio, M.J., The effects of captopril (SQ 14,225) on vascular tissue renin in spontaneously hypertensive (SHR) and WKY-normotensive (NTR) rats: Relationship to systolic blood pressure (SBP) and plasma renin activity (PRA), Pharmacologist, 21, 212, 1979.

164. Aoki, K., Experimental studies on the relationship between endocrine organs and hypertension in spontaneously hypertensive rats. III. Role of the endocrine organs and hormones, Jap. Heart J., 5, 57, 1964.

165. Okamoto, K. and Aoki, K., Development of a strain of spontaneously hypertensive rats, Jap. Circ. J., 27, 282, 1963.

166. Swales, J.D., Antagonists, inhibitors and antisera in the evaluation of vascular renin activity. In: Progress in Biochemical Pharmacology. Vol. 12: Drugs Affecting the Renin-Angiotensin-Aldosterone System. Use of Angiotensin Inhibitors, edited by G.S. Stokes and K.D.G. Edwards, pp. 98-113, S. Karger, New York.

166a Antonaccio, M.J., Rubin, B., and Horovitz, Z.P., Effects of captopril in animal models of hypertension, Clin. Exp. Hypertension, In press.

167. Margolius, H.S., Geller, R., DeJong, W., Pisano, J.J., and Sjoerdsma, A., Altered urinary kallikrein excretion in rats with hypertension, Circ. Res. 30, 358, 1972.

168. Waeber, B., Brunner, H.R., Turini, G.A., Curtet, N., and Gavras, H., Blood pressure control by captopril despite intermittent normalization of angiotensin converting enzyme activity, Clin. Res., 27, 319A, 1979.

169. McCarthy, D.A., Potter, D.E., and Nicolaides, E.D., An *in vivo* estimation of of the potencies and half-lives of synthetic bradykinin and kallidin, J. Pharmacol. Exp. Ther., 148, 117, 1965.

2. THE PHARMACOLOGY AND POTENTIAL CLINICAL APPLICATIONS OF SOMATOSTATIN AND ITS ANALOGUES

J.E. Gerich

I. Background...56

II. General Distributions and Actions...58

III. Mechanism of Action...72

IV. Metabolism...77

V. Physiologic Role of Endogenous Somatostatin...77

VI. Regulation of Pancreatic Somatostatin Secretion in Vitro...79
A. Substrates 79; B. Ionic Milieu 81; C. Neurotransmitters and other Monoamines 83; D. Hormones 86; E. Pancreatic D Cell Function in Diabetes 87.

VII. Therapeutic Potential of Somatostatin in Diabetes Mellitus and other Disorders...89

VIII. Structure-Activity Relationships: Analogues...93

References...99

I. BACKGROUND

Somatostatin was discovered in 1971, by Guillemin and his colleagues during their search for the hypothalamic growth hormone-releasing factor. A peptide was found in ovine hypothalamus which inhibited the release of growth hormone from cultured anterior pituitary cells.[1,2] Determination of its amino acid sequence[3] indicated that it was a tetradecapeptide with a molecular weight of 1639 (Figure 1). An identical peptide was later isolated from porcine hypothalamus by Schally and his coworkers.[4] The peptide was named somatostatin in the belief that it was a hypothalamic releasing factor whose sole function was to inhibit the secretion of growth hormone. It soon became evident, however, that a peptide with identical immunologic characteristics and biologic activity was present in the D cells of pancreatic islets, in D-like cells of the gastrointestinal tract, in parafollicular cells of the thyroid gland, and in extrahypothalamic neurons of both the central and peripheral nervous system in various species, including man. Moreover, studies employing synthetic somatostatin[5] demonstrated that the peptide possessed a wide spectrum of biologic activities in addition to its inhibition of growth hormone.

```
S O M A T O S T A T I N

1   2   3   4   5   6   7

Ala-Gly-Cys-Lys-Asn-Phe-Phe
        |               |
        S               Trp  8
        |               |
        S               Lys  9
        |               |
        Cys-Ser-Thr-Phe-Thr

         14  13  12  11  10
```

FIG. 1: Structure of somatostatin

II. GENERAL DISTRIBUTION AND ACTIONS

Somatostatin is widely distributed within both the central and peripheral nervous systems and in various other tissues (Table 1).[2,6-28] It is found in highest concentration in the median eminence and pancreatic islets; the largest amounts of somatostatin are found in the cerebral cortex, spinal cord, brain stem, and hypothalamus in the central nervous system, and in the portions of the stomach, thyroid, and pancreas. Lesser amounts of somatostatin have been reported in dorsal root ganglia and sympathetic ganglia (inferior and superior mesenteric, para-aortic, and superior cervical) in the guinea pig and rat,[29] and also in Auerbach's plexus of the rat intestine.[30] Somatostatin immunoreactivity which behaves chromatographically similar to synthetic somatostatin has been found in human cerebrospinal fluid[31,32] and urine;[33] increased amounts of cerebrospinal fluid somatostatin are present in various neurologic disorders (e.g. nerve root compression, spinal cord, and cerebral disease) suggesting that increases in cerebrospinal fluid levels may be a nonspecific index of brain damage.[31]

Consistent with the view that somatostatin located at extrahypothalamic sites in the nervous system may function as a neurotransmitter, the peptide has been found to alter neuronal function in various parts of the central nervous system and to modify behavior in experimental animals (Table 2).[34-44] In man, somatostatin administered intravenously has a mild tranquilizing action but no other major behavorial or motor effects.[45-47]

TABLE 1

DISTRIBUTION OF SOMATOSTATIN IN THE RAT

	Patel and Reichlin[9]			Arimura et al[10]		Kronheim et al[8]	
	ng/region	ng/mg wet wt	ng/mg/protein	ng/mg wet wt	ng/mg protein	mg/mg/wet wt	ng/mg protein
CNS structures							
Hypothalamus	77	2.3	26.1	2.12		1.10	216.4
Median Eminence			248.0		309.1		
Ventromedial Nucleus		0.44	17.5		14.6		
Brain Stem	128	0.67	5.1	0.05		0.13	53.4
Spinal cord	317	0.08	10.4			0.45	165.2
Olfactory lobe	7	0.52	1.1	0.02		0.15	21.2
Cerebral cortex	516	0.03	6.7	0.03	2.4	0.09	35.7
Cerebellum	7		0.4	0.02		0.04	28.4
Pineal			0.1		0.5		0
Pituitary							
Anterior		0					
Posterior			5.6				
Gut and visceral structures							
Stomach	306	0.37	2.4	0.17	11.7	Body of Stomach	1.6
Pylorus	116	0.52	6.4	0.43	9.7	Antrum of Stomach	20.2
Duodenum	42	0.15	1.9	0.03	1.6		2.1
Jejunum (10 cm)	50	0.07	1.9	0.03	1.6		2.3
Pancreas (whole)	137	0.17	1.8	0.14	33.8		26.4
Pancreatitis islets			786.0				
Liver			0		0		0.1
Lung			0		0		0
Kidney			0		0		0.2
Submandibular glands			0				

TABLE 2

ACTIONS OF SOMATOSTATIN ON THE NERVOUS SYSTEM

Depresses discharge frequency of neurons in cerebral cortex, cerebellar cortex, spinal cord, and ventromedial hypothalamic nucleus after micro-ontophoretic application *in vivo*[36,37].

Increases glutamine-stimulated calcium uptake and reduces calcium efflux from guinea pig cerebral synaptosomes *in vitro*[38].

Induces stereotyped behavior, alterations of sleep-wake cycle, ataxia, cataonia, convulsions, and catalepsia in rats after intraventricular administration[39,40].

Lower LD_{50} for phenobarbital, increases LD_{50} for strychnine in rats after intravenous administration[41].

Decreases firing of brain stem reticular formation neurons, reduces motor activity and alters behavior in rats after intrapentoneal administration[42,43].

Inhibits electrically stimulated acetylcholine release from guinea pig ileum myenteric plexus[44].

There is extensive evidence that hypothalamic somatostatin released from nerve terminals into the pituitary portal vasculature acts as a physiologic regulator of growth hormone and perhaps also of thyrotropin (TSH) secretion. Release of somatostatin from hypothalamic neural elements is stimulated by potassium, dopamine, and norepinephrine, and is calcium dependent.[48-50] Somatostatin does not affect posterior pituitary hormone secretion. The peptide inhibits growth hormone release at concentrations as low as 10^{-9} M *in vitro* and is also a potent inhibitor of growth hormone secretion *in vivo*. Abnormally elevated circulating growth hormone levels found in acromegaly,[51-56] poorly-controlled diabetes,[45,57,58] protein malnutrition,[56], and Laron dwarfism[59] are decreased during intravenous infusion of somatostatin. As with other *in vivo* affects of the peptide, its suppression of serum growth hormone levels is short lived (half-life 2 minutes), and after discontinuation of the somatostatin infusion, a rebound of growth hormone levels above original values is usually observed. When administered intramuscularly,[53] subcutaneously in oil,[53] or as a protamine conjugate,[60] somatostatin still has a relatively short biologic half-life (60-90 minutes). The observations in experimental animals 1) that administration of antiserum against somatostatin augments circulating growth hormone levels[61-63] and prevents stress and starvation induced suppression of serum growth hormone levels,[63,64] 2) that serum growth hormone levels are increased in baboons actively immunized against somatostatin,[65] and 3) that the decrease in hypothalamic somatostatin content observed following hypophysectomy is restored by growth hormone administration[66-69] provide convincing evidence that somatostatin released into the hypothalamic pituitary portal vessels acts as a physiologic regulator of growth hormone secretion.

Somatostatin is also a potent inhibitor of TSH secretion both in vivo and in vitro; in man, somatostatin inhibits serum TSH responses to thyrotropin releasing factor[51,70-72] and decreases both nocturnally elevated serum TSH levels in normal individuals[73] and the elevated serum TSH levels of hypothyroid patients.[74] Whether it acts as a physiologic modulator of TSH secretion is unclear at the present time but observations that systemic administration of antiserum against somatostatin augments basal serum TSH levels and TSH responses to both cold exposure and thyrotropin releasing factor in the rat[62,75-77] suggest that it might. In normal man somatostatin does not affect circulating prolactin,[51,71,72,78,79] adrenocorticotropin,[51,53,78,80] lutenizing hormone,[51,78] or follicle stimulating hormone[51,78] levels. However, in certain patients with acromegaly[55] and in cultured rat pituicytes,[82,83] somatostatin has been reported to inhibit prolactin secretion. Moreover, in patients with hypersecretion of adrenocorticotropin due to pituitary tumors (Nelson-Salassa syndrome) or during suboptimal corticosteroid replacement for Addison's disease,[81,84,85] somatostatin decreases circulating adrenocorticotropin hormone levels.

In human, rat, and dog thyroid, somatostatin has been localized immunohistochemically to cells lining thyroid follicles.[10,24-26] Somatostatin does not affect parathyroid hormone secretion[86] but has been reported to decrease serum calcitonin levels in patients with medullary carcinoma of the thyroid.[87] There are conflicting data concerning thyroid hormone release; in mice whose thyroids had been prelabeled with I-125, somatostatin has been reported to decrease the appearance of I-125 in blood after administration of thyrotropin.[88] In man, somatostatin has no consistent effects on serum triiodothyronine (T_3) and tetraiodothyronine (T_4) increments after thyrotropin administration.[89,90]

In the gastrointestinal tract, somatostatin is found in D-like cells in stomach, duodenum, jejunum, and salivary glands,[2,6,8-10,19,23,91-95] in saliva,[91] gastric juice,[96,96] duodenal aspirates,[98,99] in neurons of Auerbach's plexus,[30] and in fibers of the vagus nerve.[100] Various gastrointestinal tract functions are affected by somatostatin: basal and stimulated secretion of gastrin,[101-109] pancreozymin,[104,110,111] vasoactive intestinal peptide,[112] gut glucagon,[113] motilin,[114] gastric inhibitory polypeptide,[115] secretin,[104,110,116,117] and pancreatic polypeptide[118,119] are inhibited by somatostatin in various species. Somatostatin also directly inhibits gastric acid, pepsin, and intrinsic factor secretion, gastric motility,[101,105,106,118-122] gall bladder contraction,[125,126,128] and both small and large intestinal motility,[129,130] absorption,[131,132] and secretion.[133] Despite these numerous effects of somatostatin on gastrointestinal function, to date no malabsorption has been reported during long-term infusions of somatostatin in man.[45]

Based on the actions described above, several potential therapeutic applications of somatostatin in gastrointestinal disorders have been suggested; somatostatin prevents the development of cysteamine-induced duodenal ulcers in rats, a model for stress-induced ulcers,[134] and has been reported to stop duodenal ulcer bleeding in man.[135] However, somatostatin did not improve the course of taurocholate-induced pancreatitis in the rat.[136]

Intra-aortic administration of somatostatin to rats has been reported to cause a prompt increase in urine flow and in free water clearance without concomitant changes in renal blood flow, osmolar clearance, electrolyte excretion, and cyclic AMP excretion.[137] In dogs, somatostatin has been shown to increase free water clearance during infusion of arginine vasopressin.[138] Since the peptide does not affect antidiuretic hormone secretion in this species,[138a] the above results can be best explained on the basis of antagonism of the action of antidiuretic hormone. In the isolated toad bladder preparation, somatostatin has been reported to antagonize the hydroosmotic effect of vasopressin and to enhance water flow induced by cAMP.[138b] However, no effect has been found on serum electrolytes, urine volume, and electrolyte balance during prolonged infusion of somatostatin in man.[45]

Increases in plasma renin activity following furosemide administration[139,140] or infusion of a beta adrenergic agonist[141] in man are decreased by somatostatin, but basal circulating plasma renin activity is not affected. These results suggest that somatostatin may inhibit secretion of renin by the kidney. Transient increases in blood pressure (5-10 mmHg) and pulse (5-10 beats/min) have been occasionally observed after bolus injection of somatostatin, but in normal man, somatostatin does not affect cardiac output, stroke volume, cardiac index, stroke index, or total peripheral resistance.[142] In individuals with moderate to severe hypertension, somatostatin has been reported to decrease blood pressure[142] and to prolong the hypotensive action of diazoxide.[143]

Administration of somatostatin usually has no effect on circulating leukocyte, erythrocyte, or platelet concentrations;[45,144-147] however, a 25 percent reduction leukocyte count has been found in patients with acute bacterial leukocytosis.[144] In baboons with chronically implanted intravenous catheters profound thrombocytopenia has been reported with infusions of large quantities of somatostatin;[148] in rats somatostatin apparently prevents pyromen and endotoxin-induced leukocytosis.[149] Diminished aggregation of platelets in baboons,[148] rabbits,[150] and man[151] has been found in some studies with somatostatin; however, most studies indicate no effect on platelet aggregation, bleeding time, prothrombin time, partial thromboplastin time, fibrinogen, fibrin split products, factor VII, and Von Willebrand factor in man.[45,145-147,152,152]

In addition to the above actions, somatostatin inhibits insulin and glucagon secretion (Figure 2).[154-167] It is as potent an inhibitor of insulin and glucagon secretion <u>in vivo</u> and <u>in vitro</u> as it is of growth hormone secretion.[154,159] The degree to which somatostatin inhibits insulin and glucagon secretion varies depending upon the dose of the peptide employed and the stimulus used for insulin and glucagon secretion. For example, <u>in vitro</u> using the perfused rat pancreas with arginine (19 mM) plus glucose (5.5 mM) as stimuli somatostatin appeared to be a more

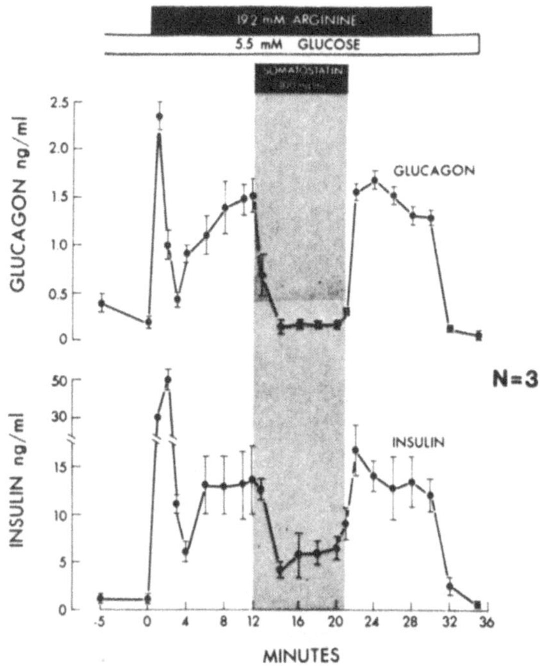

FIG. 2: Somatostatin inhibition of arginine-stimulated insulin and glucagon release from the perfused rat pancreas.[160]

effective inhibitor of glucagon release than of insulin release.[160] In contrast, under other conditions, insulin release appears to be more sensitive to somatostatin inhibition than is glucagon secretion.[161-163]

The response of insulin and glucagon to all known secretagogues can be inhibited by an appropriate concentration of somatostatin; among these are orciprenaline,[178] glucose,[160,176-185] glucagon,[186-189] arginine[161,175 184,185,190-192] secretin,[186] theophylline,[160,176,181] tolbutamide,[177,181, 187,189] isoproterenol,[160,186] calcium,[161,181,193] potassium,[176] epinephrine[194-196] meals,[45,197-200] 3-isobutyl-methyl-xanthine,[193] the divalent ionophore A23187,[193,201] cyclic AMP,[188] and dibutyryl cyclic AMP.[202] Onset of inhibition is virtually immediate and is reversible upon withdrawl of somatostatin. In general, increasing the concentration of a given secretagogue can overcome the inhibitory effect of a given dose of somatostatin as in the case of glucose[181,189] and calcium.[161] Of interest is the observation that in vitro, the first phase of glucose-stimulated insulin appears to be 25-50 times more sensitive to inhibition by somatostatin than is the second phase.[179]

The ability of somatostatin to inhibit insulin and glucagon secretion and its presence in pancreatic islets suggests that this peptide may be important in regulating insulin and glucagon secretion. This concept is supported by studies showing that under appropriate conditions, antiserum against somatostatin can augment glucagon[203] and insulin[203a,204] release from isolated pancreatic islets. Presently, it seems that locally released somatostatin rather than circulating somatostatin would be involved in this process since neither active[65] nor passive immunization[205] of animals against somatostatin alters circulating insulin and glucagon levels.

Somatostatin has been used in a variety of metabolic studies *in vivo*.[45,51,52,57,58,79,80,132,159,186,187,191,195-200,206-261] At doses used *in vivo*, somatostatin has no direct effect on hepatic, adipose, or muscle tissue;[213,262,263] thus the acute alterations in carbohydrate, lipid, and amino acid metabolism observed during administration of somatostatin *in vivo* have been attributed to the effects of somatostatin on hormone secretion-mainly those of suppressing insulin, glucagon, and growth hormone secretion. However, effects that occur *in vivo* with somatostatin are dose dependent since by varying the dose one can modify the extent to which insulin and glucagon secretion are suppressed. Measurement of peripheral circulating levels of insulin and glucagon might not accurately reflect the relative extent to which the secretion of each hormone has been suppressed since the hepatic extraction of each is different and may be altered by somatostatin.[214]

When somatostatin is infused in normal humans and other species at doses in excess of 200 ng/kg/min, fasting plasma glucose levels decline 20-30 percent over the initial hour[215-224] and then increase to values 20-30 percent above control levels;[215,221,223] this delayed hyperglycemia occurs despite the persistent suppression of insulin, glucagon, and growth hormone secretion. This is due to a decrease in glucose production exceeding a concomitant decrease in glucose utilization[223] which can be attributed to suppression of insulin secretion by somatostatin since sustained hypoglycemia occurs when somatostatin is infused along with replacement amounts of insulin.[264] Infusion of somatostatin along with replacement amounts of glucagon results in marked hyperglycemia.[215,217] With prolonged infusions of somatostatin at lower doses (60 ng/kg/min),[225] a variable decrease in plasma glucose levels occurs and no sustained increase above fasting levels is observed. Thus, at this dose, somatostatin does not cause fasting hyperglycemia. In hyperglycemic insulin-dependent diabetes infusion of somatostatin at a dose of 500 μg/hr causes a sustained and progressive decrease in circulating glucose levels for as long as six hours;[226] the hyperglycemia and hyperketonemia occurring after acute withdrawal of insulin can be markedly decreased (Figure 3).[57] The above results have been interpreted to indicate that both insulin and glucagon are important in normal glucose homeostasis and that somatostatin suppression of glucagon secretion can mollify the acute metabolic consequences of insulin deficiency.[228] In insulin-dependent (maturity-onset type) diabetics not being treated with insulin, infusion of somatostatin may increase or not improve pre-existing fasting hyperglycemia;[229,230] this is probably due to suppression of insulin release since infusion of somatostatin in maturity-onset diabetics being treated with insulin decreases fasting hyperglycemia.[45] In normal man, somatostatin enhances the hypoglycemic action of exogenous insulin.[80,224,231]

Increases in plasma glucose during infusions of alanine,[241] arginine,[206,249] and epinephrine[195,196] are diminished or prevented by somatostatin, suggesting that the increase in plasma glucose normally seen under

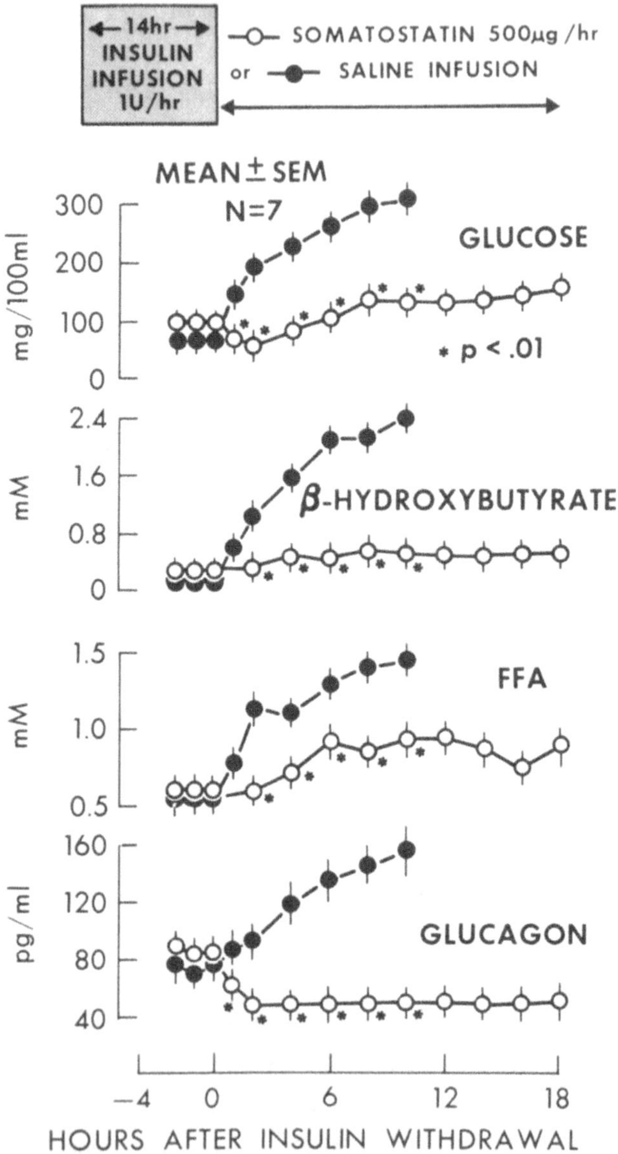

FIG. 3: Effect of somatostatin infusion on development of hyperglycemia and hyperketonemia after withdrawal of insulin from insulin-dependent diabetics.[57]

these conditions are primarily mediated through stimulation of glucagon secretion. Glucose responses to exogenous glucagon[186,187,189,215] or the beta adrenergic agent oxyprenaline[178] are increased during infusion of somatostatin; this is probably due to concomitant inhibition of insulin secretion by somatostatin. Decreases in plasma glucose following insulin administration are augmented by somatostatin:[80,224,231] since this is reversed by concomitant infusion of glucagon along with somatostatin,[80] these studies have provided evidence for a role for glucagon as an acute counterregulatory hormone.

In normal man, hyperglycemia seen after oral or intravenous glucose administration and after meal ingestion is augmented during infusion of somatostatin due to its inhibition of insulin secretion;[184,189,200,233,235,237] in insulin-dependent juvenile diabetics and in adult-onset diabetics receiving exogenous insulin, hyperglycemia seen after meals or glucose ingeston is decreased.[45,58,197,200,237] In adult-onset diabetics not being treated with insulin, administration of somatostatin exaggerates postprandial hyperglycemia.[183,199,230,234,237] The improvement in glucose tolerance seen in juvenile-onset diabetics and adult-onset diabetics receiving exogenous insulin has been attributed to suppression of glucagon secretion and to interference with glucose absorption. The latter appears to exert a minor effect, however, since improvement in postprandial hyperglycemia in insulin-trated diabetics following ingestion of carbohydrate free diets has been observed.[233]

Variable effects of somatostatin have been observed on other substrates. In normal man free fatty acid[222,229] and glycerol[222] levels have been reported to increase during infusion of somatostatin whereas, in insulin treated diabetics no change[236,242] or a decrease[244] have been found. Increments in circulating fatty acid levels during stimulation of lipolysis by epinephrine[196] are not affected by somatostatin but responses to oxyprenalol[178] are augmented. In adult-onset diabetics[229] fasting ketone body levels increase slightly during infusion of somatostatin, whereas in juvenile-onset diabetics[236,244] withdrawn from insulin no change or a decrease has been found. Plasma lactate levels are not affected by somatostatin but the lactate responses to administration of epinephrine are increased.[195] During infusion of somatostatin, plasma branched chain amino acids are alanine have been reported to increase slightly[211,222,229] or to remain unchanged.[215] Splanchnic uptake of amino acids decreases almost 50 percent during infusion of somatostatin (probably due to inhibition of glucagon secretion); this is paralleled by a decrease in net splanchnic glucose output.[215] Leucine turnover has been reported to be decreased in man during infusion of somatostatin.[211]

III. MECHANISM OF ACTION

It is generally assumed that somatostatin acts by a similar mechanism in the various tissues in which it acts. The most extensively studied action of somatostatin has been its inhibition of pancreatic islet hormone secretion. The onset of somatostatin action is rapid and does not depend on protein synthesis[2,265,266] suggesting that it may act like other peptide hormones via an interaction with plasma membrane receptors rather than like steroid or thyroid hormones which require intracellular translocation and are dependent on protein synthesis. High-affinity binding sites for somatostatin have been identified in cultured anterior pituitary cells[267] and on partially purified plasma membranes of pituicytes[268] and pancratic B cells (Figure 4).[268,269] Some of these tissues, however, were derived from tumors and thus characteristics of these receptors may not necessarily reflect those of normal tissue. The binding affinity for somatostatin receptors on cultured pituicytes is approximately 1 x 10^{10} M^{-1} and it has been estimated that these cells contain approximately 14,000 binding sites.[267] These observatons and the fact that somatostatin inhibits both neuronal[34,35] and pancratic B cell[270] electrical activity suggest a plasma membrane site of action for somatostatin. However, additional loci of action may be operative since cytosolic somatostatin binding proteins have been found in several tissues[271] and since somatostatin has been reported to inhibit cyclic AMP stimulated protein kinase activity in secretory vesicles of isolated pancreatic islets and pituicytes.[272]

There is considerable evidence that calcium is involved in stimulus-secretion coupling in both endocrine and exocrine systems:[273] Extracellular calcium is essential for secretion in both systems; during stimulation of insulin release by glucose pancreatic islets take up calcium from the extracellular fluid and decrease islet calcium release.[274] Moreover, increasing extracellular concentrations within the physiologic range augments insulin release.[275] Observations that elevation of extracellular calcium

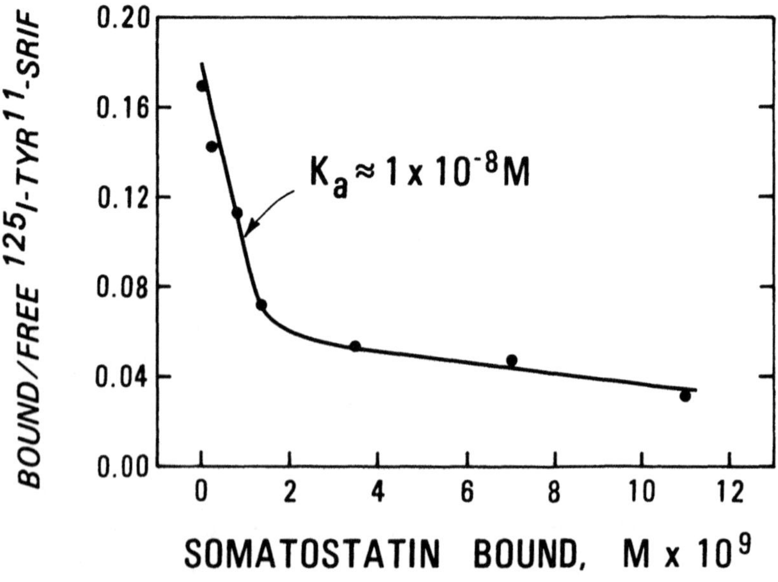

FIG. 4: Scatchard plot of somatostatin binding to purified plasma membranes of human insulinoma *(R. Rizza and J. Gerich, unpublished observations).*

concentration[161,181,276,277] and the addition of the divalent cation ionophore A23187[277,278] or theophylline[277,288] (which may mobilize intracellular calcium) can at least partly reverse somatostatin inhibition of insulin secretion suggest that somatostatin might act by intervening with cellular calcium fluxes or with an action of calcium. Initial reports of the diminution of pancreatic islet[161,279] and pituitary cell[280] calcium uptake durig somatostatin inhibition of the release of their respective hormones supported this concept. However, some of these results have not been subsequently confirmed.[281,282] Moreover, somatostatin has been shown to inhibit insulin,[200] glucagon,[193] and growth hormone[283] secretion stimulated by the calcium ionophore A23187 in the presence of low extracellular calcium and also to inhibit insulin release stimulated by isobutylmethylxanthine in the absence of extracellular calcium.[283]

Another potential mechanism by which somatostatin may inhibit hormone secretion is by interference with cellular cyclic nucleotide metabolism since cyclic nucleotides, particularly cyclic 3',5' adenosine monophosphate (cyclic AMP), are well known to be important in endocrine and exocrine secretion.[273] Indeed, somatostatin has been reported to decrease cyclic AMP levels in pituitary[284,285] and pancreatic islets.[286-288] However, several observations suggest that somatostatin may not inhibit secretion by lowering tissue cyclic AMP levels: Firstly, somatostatin inhibits growth hormone response to prostaglandin E_2 and isobutylmethylxanthine without affecting pituitary cyclic AMP, cyclic GMP, or protein kinase responses.[289] Secondly, somatostatin can inhibit glucagon-stimulated insulin release without affecting glucation activation of adenylate cyclase;[188] thirdly, somatostatin inhibits insulin and glucagon responses to arginine[160] which apparently stimulates islet hormone secretion by a mechanism independent of cyclic AMP;[290] fourthly, somatostatin uniformly blocks hormone responses to agents which increase tissue cyclic AMP levels by different means, e.g. adenylate cyclase activation[160] and phosphodiesterase inhibition;[160] and lastly, somatostatin inhibits pituitary and pancreatic hormone secretion in response to exogenous cyclic AMP and its analogues.[188,202,277] The reported action of somatostatin on cyclic AMP levels may represent a nonspecific pharmacologic effect since it has been reported to occur in tissues which do not possess specific somatostatin receptors. Somatostatin does not increase islet phosphodiesterase activity[291] or affect islet sodium-potassium ATPase activity[292] in pancreatic islet tissue. Thus, rather than acting through an alteration of cellular cyclic AMP levels, somatostatin may act by interfering with cyclic nucleotide action perhaps at a site where cyclic nucleotide-calcium interaction is involved. It has been suggested that somatostatin may inhibit insulin and glucagon secretion through an alpha adrenergic receptor mechanism.[293,294] However, several _in vivo_ and _in vitro_ studies have shown that doses of phentolamine (an alpha adrenergic receptor antagonist) which reverse inhibition of insulin release due to epinephrine have no effect on inhibition of insulin release due to somatostatin.[295-298]

IV. METABOLISM

The half-life of exogenously infused somatostatin is about 1-2 minutes in man and dogs.[299,300] Its metabolic clearance rate (≈ 30 ml/kg/min in normal man) is unaffected by liver disease but is decreased in patients with chronic renal failure, suggesting that the kidney may play a role in the metabolism of somatostatin.[300] Arteriovenous differences in somatostatin levels during infusion of the peptide in baboons and rats indicate that tissues such as liver, muscle, and kidney may be major sites of degradation.[301,302] Crude brain and hypothalamic extracts,[303-305] isolated guinea pig pancreatic islet cells,[306] perfused rat pancreas,[306] and both rat and human serum degrade synthetic somatostatin.[307] Rat serum contains both an aminopeptidase and an endopeptidase which appear to be involved in degrading somatostatin.[307] Peptidases present in brain extracts cleave the amino terminal alanine and glycine residues and also the internal residues (Phe^{6}-Phe^{7}, Trp^{8}--Lys^{9}, Thr^{9},-Phe^{10}).[303] Induction of hypothyroidism has been reported to decrease degradation of somatostatin by rat hypothalamus;[308] conceivably decreased degradation of somatostatin might explain the increased concentrations of somatostatin found in the pancreas and other tissues of hypothyroid and hypophysectomized rats.[309]

V. PHYSIOLOGIC ROLE OF ENDOGENOUS SOMATOSTATIN

Four functions for somatostatin have been proposed depending on its location: a neurotransmitter, a neurohormone, a parahormone, and a hormone. The location of somatostatin in extrahypothalamic neurons in the central nervous system, the biological actions of somatostatin on behavior and neuronal function, and the release of somatostatin from synaptosomes by agents such as dopamine and norepinephrine provide considerable evidence that somatostatin may function as a peptidergic <u>neurotransmitter</u>. There is also considerable evidence that somatostatin most likely acts as a <u>neurohormone</u> regulating the secretion of growth hormone and thyrotropin; namely, the peptide is present in hypothalamic neurons of the median eminence; it is released into the hypophyseal portal vessels; it is a potent inhibitor of all known stimuli for growth hormone and thyrotropin release; its hypothalamic concentration is altered by hypophysectomy, growth hormone administration, and hypothyroidism; and, finally, its neutralization by either passive or active immunization increases growth hormone and thyrotropin secretin.

The location of somatostatin in the mucosa of the gastrointestinal tract and in pancreatic islets and the ability of exogenous somatostatin to alter the function of adjacent cells in these locations suggest that endogenous somatostatin may play a role in the regulation of gastrointestinal and pancreatic islet function. The failure of active immunization and passive immunization to alter insulin and glucagon secretion *in vivo* whereas direct application of antisomatostatin serum to pancreatic islets *in vitro* can increase insulin and/or glucagon release suggest that, at least with respect to pancreatic islets, endogenous somatostatin probably acts as a local regulator (<u>parahormone</u>) rather than as a classical hormone which must traverse through the circulation prior to acting at its target.

VI. REGULATION OF PANCREATIC SOMATOSTATIN SECRETION IN VITRO

To date, only a few studies have examined secretion or release of somatostatin from tissues other than the pancreas; therefore, in the subsequent section, only studies[310-335] of secretion of pancreatic somatostatin will be reviewed.

A. Substrates

Glucose stimulates biphasic release of somatostatin from the perfused dog,[315,334] rat,[318] and cat pancreas and from perfused rat islets (Figure 5).[314,325] Both phases of somatostatin release coincide with corresponding phases of insulin release.

The magnitude of both phases of somatostatin responses to glucose appear to be less than those of insulin regardless of species studied[314,315,318,325] but no dose-response studies have been performed comparing each phase of somatostatin and insulin responses to glucose.

To what extent stimulation of somatostatin secretion by glucose is dependent upon metabolism of glucose is unclear. Galactose, which is not metabolized by islets and which does not stimulate insulin release has been reported not to cause release of somatostatin from neonatal rat islet monolayers.[329] Mannoheptulose, a blocker of glucose phosphorylation in islets, which inhibits glucose-stimulated insulin release, has been reported to inhibit glucose-stimulated somatostatin release from incubated rat islets.[311] These

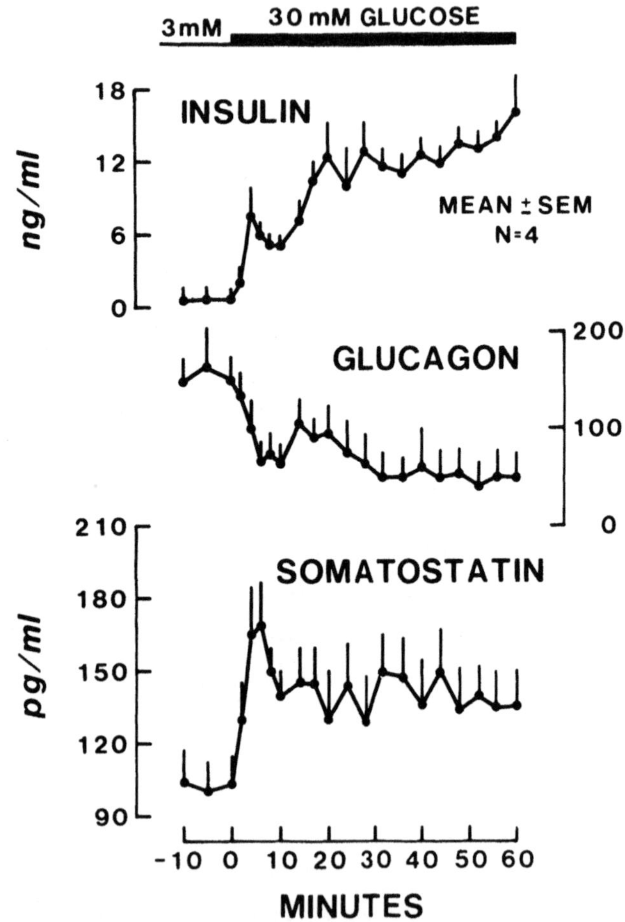

FIG. 5: Effect of glucose on insulin, glucagon and somatostatin release from rat islets perfused *in vitro (M. Itch and J. Gerich, unpublished observations).*

results could be due to either the fact that a substrate-stimulus must be metabolized in order to stimulate somatostatin release or that an energy source must be available for somatostatin secretion to occur. Of great interest is the observation that D-glyceraldehyde, a metabolite of glucose, inhibits somatostatin release (while stimulating insulin release) from incubated rat islets;[314] this represents the first instance of a dissociation between somatostatin and insulin release and would suggest that stimulation of somatostatin release by glucose may not simply be the direct consequence of the metabolism of glucose. The effects of carbohydrates other than glucose, galactose, and D-glyceraldehyde on somatostatin release have not been examined.

Arginine,[312,312,318,323,324,332-334] leucine,[315,316] and the metabolite of leucine, α-ketoisocaproic acid[316] have been demonstrated to stimulate somatostatin release in several systems. In perfusion systems such as the perfused cat pancreas (Figure 6) both arginine and leucine cause biphasic somatostatin release when superimposed upon a background of basal (2-5 mM) glucose. Whether arginine in the absence of glucose would stimulate somatostatin release has not been established.

B. Ionic Milieu

It is well established that the ionic composition of the extracellular fluid exerts an important influence on both insulin and

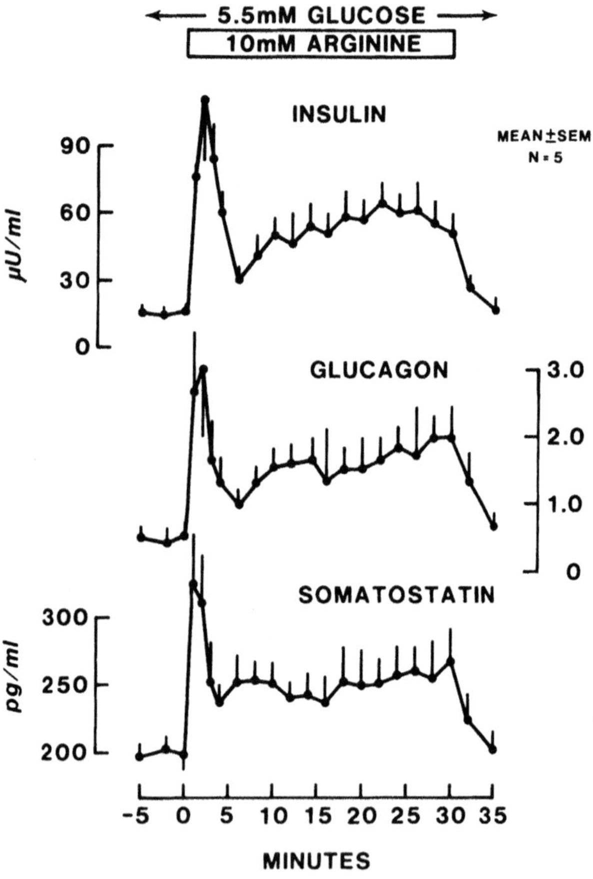

FIG. 6: Stimulation of biphasic secretion of insulin, glucagon and somatostatin from the cat pancreas perfused *in vitro*. (*J. Gerich, unpublished observations*).

glucagon release. The presence of extracellular calcium is essential for release of both insulin and glucagon and that, over a given range, increases in the extracellular calcium or potassium concentrations increase insulin release while increases in the extracellular magnesium concentrations decrease insulin release. The effects of extracellular ionic milieu on somatostatin secretion have not been studied in detail as of yet. It appears that like insulin and glucagon release, secretion of somatostatin from the pancreas requires the presence of extracellular calcium and is increased by increasing the extracellular calcium concentration.[334] Release of somatostatin from rat cerebral cortex,[336] neurohypophysis,[337] and hypothalamus[338] has also been shown to be calcium dependent.

C. Neurotransmitters and other Monoamines

The effects of catecholamines and monoamines on somatostatin release from the pancreas and neural tissue have been investigated by several groups.[311,321,325,333,339-341]

Epinephrine inhibits release of somatostatin from the pancreas (Figure 7). In an in-depth study employing the perfused dog pancreas, Samols et al[326] examined the effects of various adrenergic agents, concluded that beta adrenergic mechanisms were responsible for increasing somatostatin release while alpha adrenergic mechanisms were responsible for inhibiting somatostatin release. This conclusion is consistent with the findings that isoproterenol augments somatostatin release[334] and that agents such as theophylline [172,174,185,186,188,190] and cAMP derivatives[168,186] increase pancreatic somatostatin release.[310,314,316,328,330,333]

Acetlycholine stimulates pancreatic somatostatin release (Figure 7).[334] Vagal stimulation causes release of somatostatin into the gastric antrum of cats.[342] Dopamine has been reported to inhibit somatostatin release from incubated rat islets by Barden et al.[321] Since dopamine - in addition to specific domaminergic actions - may also have, depending on the concentration used, alpha and beta adrenergic actions as well, it is unclear whether this action of dopamine is dopaminergic or adrenergic. Of interest is the report of Uvnas-Wallensten et al.[343] that apomorphine, a relatively specific dopaminergic agonist, increases somatostatin release into the gastric antrum of cats. Others have found that dopamine increases the release of somatostatin from rat hypothalamus.[340,341,344] Also, norepinephrine[341,344] and acetylcholine[341] increase somatostatin release from rat hypothalamus. The discrepancy between the effects of dopamine (stomach and pancreas) and norepinephrine (hypothalamus and pancreas) on somatostatin release in different tissues is not unique since opposite effect of these agents have been reported on somatostatin release from synapotosomes from different parts of the brain (cerebral cortex and hypothalamus).[339] Serotonin has been reported to increase release of

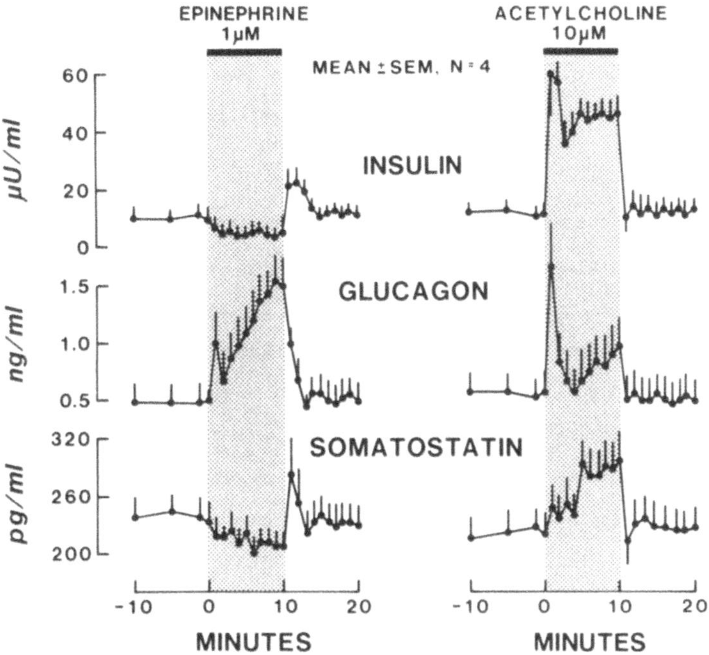

FIG. 7: Effect of epinephrine and acetylcholine on release of insulin, glucagon and somatostatin from the perfused cat pancreas (*J. Gerich, unpublished observations*).

somatostatin from both rat hypothalamic and cerebral cortex synaptosomes.[339] No studies have as yet been performed examining the effect of this monoamine on pancreatic somatostatin release.

D. Hormones

Various peptide hormones have been shown to alter pancratic somatostatin secretion: glucagon,[313,316,321,324,326,335] pancreozymin,[315] gastrin,[317] secretin,[317] gastric inhibitory polypeptide,[319] all stimulate somatostatin release. B-endorphin, an opioid peptide, (and morphine) inhibits somatostatin release from the perfused dog pancreas[320] while neurotensin stimulates somatostatin release from isolated rat islets at low glucose concentrations (3 mM) but inhibits somatostatin responses at 23 mM glucose or 20 mM arginine.[332] The physiologic significance of the above observations are unclear since in virtually all instances what would be considered pharmacologic doses of each hormone were employed. However, based on the observation that all the gastrointestinal hormones studied increased somatostatin secretion, the fact that exogenous somatostatin inhibits the release of each of these hormones, and finally, the fact that somatostatin is found in the gastrointestinal tract, it has been proposed that gastrointestinal somatostatin may act in some feedback inhibition axis to regulate nutrient absorption.

Although ability of physiologic concentrations of glucagon to augment pancreatic somatostatin has not been demonstrated, the recent report that somatostatin release from islet monolayers is augmented by antiglucagon serum[329] strongly suggests that glucagon may play a physiologic role in the regulation of islet D cell function. Conceivably, the prolonged hyperglucagonemia associated with alloxan diabetes may explain in part the D cell hyperplasia and increased somatostatin release from pancreases of alloxan diabetic rats perfused *in vitro*.[323] No studies have been able to demonstrate an acute effect of insulin in mammalian islet somatostatin release.

E. Pancreatic D Cell Function in Diabetes

Abnormalities in islet D cell morphology in human diabetes and in alloxan diabetes in the rat were reported more than 25 years ago using conventional histochemical methods.[345-350] Recently, using more sophisticated immunohistochemical and radioimmunoassay techniques, it has been confirmed that spontaneous and induced diabetes causes significant changes in islet D cells. In rats with alloxan- and streptozotocin-induced diabetes there is an increase in the number of islet D cells and in the content of pancreatic or islet somatostatin which is associated with a decrease in the number of islet B cells and in the content of pancreatic or islet insulin.[240,241,244] These types of diabetes are characterized by hypoinsulinemia and hyperglucagonemia *in vivo*.

In the only study to date directly examining secretion of somatostatin in alloxan diabetes;[323] in this study, it was found that two weeks after induction of alloxan diabetes in rats - a time at which pancreatic somatostatin content should still be normal - there was excessive release of somatostatin from pancreases perfused in vitro during arginine stimulation; this was accompanied by markedly decreased insulin and slightly decreased glucagon responses. These results indicate that D cell function is abnormal in alloxan diabetes, that it may precede gross changes in D cell mass, and that it may contribute to concommitant abnormalities of insulin and glucagon release.

In contrast to the above insulinopenic types of induced diabetes, that caused by the M variant of the encephalomyocarditis virus results in a decrease in islet D cells along with decreases in islet B cells and increases in islet A cells.[351] A similar decreased pancreatic somatostatin content associated with decreased insulin and increased glucagon content has been found in the spontaneously diabetic Chinese hamster.[352] This animal, in contrast to most other widely studied animals with spontaneous diabetes, is not obese. The importance of the decrease in islet somatostatin content and islet D cell number to the abnormalities of insulin and glucagon release in the above two animal models of diabetes is unclear, since there are no studies of somatostatin secretion in either of these models.

Variable changes in pancreatic or islet somatostatin content have been found in other closely related models of spontaneous diabetes

- OBOB and DBDB mice.[353,354] Decreased pancreatic somatostatin content or decreased numbers of islet D cells increases in the number of D cells or in pancreatic somatostatin content have been found. Reasons for these discrepancies have not been completely resolved although factors related to differences in the ages of the animals studies and the severity of their diabetes have been suggested as possible explanations.

VII. THERAPEUTIC POTENTIAL OF SOMATOSTATIN IN DIABETES MELLITUS AND OTHER DISORDERS

Table 3 lists some disorders in which somatostatin or one of its analogues may be of potential therapeutic use. The ability of the peptide to inhibit renin, ACTH, growth hormone, gastrin, VIP, insulin and glucagon secretion could conceivably be put to use in the treatment of conditions resulting from excessive secretion of these hormones where alternative modes of therapy are not effective or are not available. The ability of somatostatin to inhibit gastric acid secretin and pancreatic enzyme release suggest a use in the management of peptic ulcer disease and acute pancreatitis. Some studies have provided evidence for beneficial effects of the peptide in these conditions.[134-136] The ability of somatostatin to decrease splanchnic blood flow[355] suggest that the peptide may be useful in the treatment of bleeding esophageal varices.[356] The ability of somatostatin to delay gastric emptying and the absorption of carbohydrates may find use in the treatment of reactive hypoglycemia and the Dumping Syndrome.

TABLE 3

DISORDERS IN WHICH THERE IS A POTENTIAL THERAPEUTIC USE OF SOMATOSTATIN OR ITS ANALOGUES.

Diabetes Mellitus	Cushing's Syndrome
Peptic Ulcer Disease	Insulinoma
Acute Pancreatitis	Glucagonoma
Gastrointestinal Hemorrhage	Dumping Syndrome
Syndrome of Inappropriate ADH Secretion	Hyperreninemic Hypertension
Zollinger-Ellison Syndrome	Neuropsychiatric Disorders
Verner Morrison Syndrome	Reactive Hypoglycemia
Acromegaly	

Antagonism by somatostatin of ADH action could find use as an adjunct in the treatment of syndromes due to the inappropriate secretion of antidiuretic hormone. Moreover, given the behavioral effects of somatostatin and its probable role as a neurotransmitter, it would not be unreasonable for it to find use in the treatment of some neuropsychiatric disorders. However, it should be pointed out that all of the above potential uses have not been subjected to systematic investigation and are mainly theoretical extrapolations of pharmacologic effects of somatostatin. In many instances, satisfactory treatment modulates are already available.

In contrast to the above, a therapeutic use of somatostatin in diabetes has been carefully and extensively examined. Short-term infusions of somatostatin decrease fasting[226,227] and postprandial[208] hyperglycemia in human diabetes and also prevent the development of severe ketoacidosis following acute withdrawal of insulin from patients with insulin-dependent diabetes.[57] These actions strongly suggest that somatostatin or some longer-acting and more selective analogue[357] may be useful as an adjunct to insulin in the metabolic management of this disorder. Because of the short duration of action of somatostatin no long-term studies have been undertaken to evaluate this possibility. However, several short-term studies ranging in duration from 24 to 72 hours[45,233,235,237] have indicated that administration of somatostatin along with insulin improves diurnal hyperglycemia to a degree not achievable with the same or greater doses of insulin alone (Figure 8). In all of these therapeutic trials no adverse

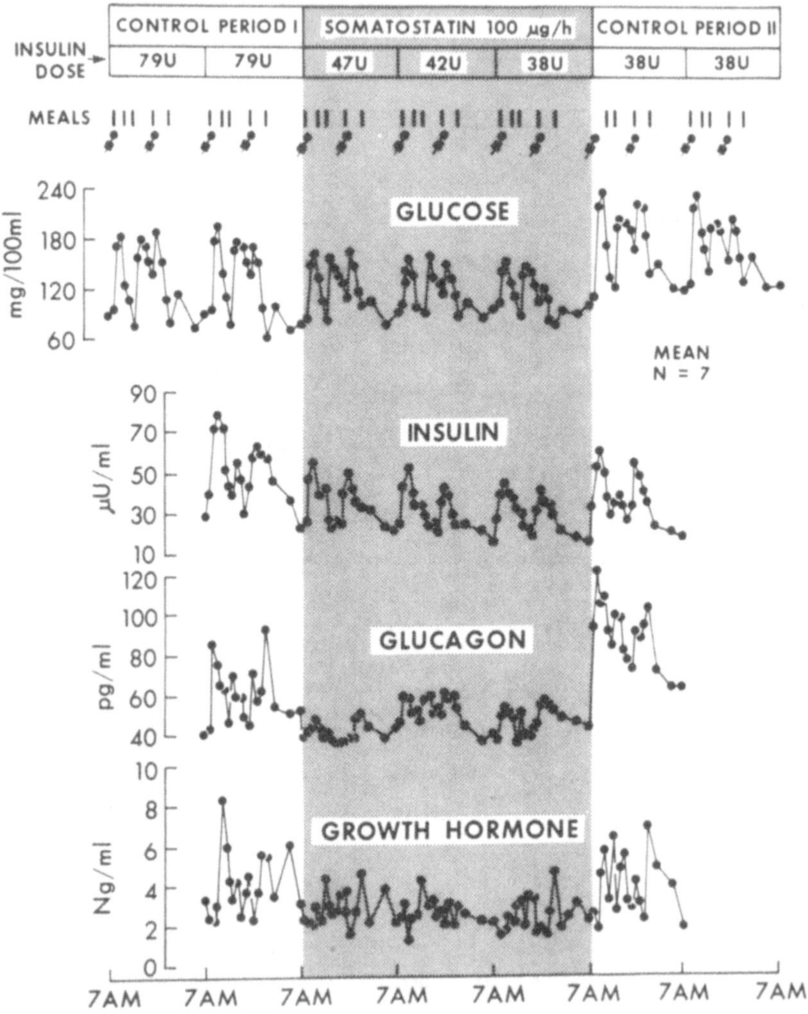

FIG. 8: Effect of three-day somatostatin infusion on diabetic control in insulin-treated juvenile and adult-onset diabetics.[45]

effects from the somatostatin infusion were observed; however, the duration of these studies has not been sufficient to exclude the emergence of adverse effects with more prolonged administration of the peptide (e.g. hypothyroidism due to inhibition of TSH secretion).

VIII. STRUCTURE-ACTIVITY RELATIONSHIPS: ANALOGUES

Synthetic somatostatin is not practical for clinical use because of its nonspecificity and short duration of action. Major efforts in several laboratories over the past five years have been directed toward the development of analogues of somatostatin with both greater specificity and longer duration of action.[164-174,312-321,358-367] The general approach to modification of the somatostatin molecule has been 1) deletion of amino acid residues; 2) substitution with other amino acids; 3) substitution with the corresponding D-amino acid; and (most commonly) 4) a combination of 1, 2 and 3.

Comparison of the biologic activities of these analogues with those of the native molecule have led to the hypothesis[173] that the hydrophobic residues (phe^6,phe^7,trp^8,phe^{11}) and the $lysine^9$ are involved in receptor binding and activation, and that $threonine^{10}$ may be an essential spacer residue while the cysteines and other amino acids determine the 3-dimensional structure[368] of the active site of the molecule. Modifications of the N-terminus do not appreciably reduce potency of the peptide: Thus des-$alanine^1$-somatostatin, N-tyrosine-somatostatin, $tyrosine^1$-somatostatin and N-tyrosine-glycine-tyrosine-somatostatin have virtually full biologic activity while des-alanine^{1}-glycine^{2}-somatostatin is 60 percent as potent as the native molecule.[173,361] Substitution of alanine for glycine^{2}, lysine^{4}, asparagine^{5}, threonine^{10}, threonine^{12}, or serine^{13} does not markedly alter biologic activity whereas replacement of phenylalanine^{6}, phenylalanine^{7}, tryptophan^{8}, lysine^{9}, or phenylalanine^{11} markedly decreases potency (Table 4).[172,173]

Both *in vivo* and *in vitro* the oxidized (cyclic) and reduced (linear) forms of somatostatin are equipotent. Whether this is due to similar intrinsic potency of the molecules or to conversion of the reduced form of the oxidized form in assay systems is unclear; analogues such as alanine^{3,14}-somatostatin and S-methionine-cysteine^{3,14}-somatostatin which cannot be cyclized have little biologic activity.[359,360] Thus, it appears that molecular conformation is important in receptor recognition of the somatostatin molecule.

Several analogues have been synthesized which possess increased potency, more prolonged duration of action or preferential effects. Substitution of the D-isomer of tryptophan for the L-isomer of tryptophan at position 8 results in an eight to tenfold increase in potency;[362] there is evidence to suggest that this is not the result of a decreased metabolism of the analogue compared to the native compound.[173] Des-aspargine^{5}-somatostatin and des-alanine^{1}, glycine^{2}-somatostatin have been reported to inhibit insulin but not glucagon secretion at appropriate concentrations whereas analogues such as D-cysteine^{14}-somatostatin, alanine^{2}-somatostatin, alanine^{2},D-cysteine^{14}-somatostatin, D-tryptophan^{8}, D-cysteine^{14}-somatostatin

TABLE 4

RELATIVE POTENCY VALUES OF SOMATOSTATIN (SRIF) AND SOMATOSTATIN ANALOGS ON INHIBITION OF GH RELEASE FROM ANTERIOR PITUITARY CELLS *IN VITRO* AND ON INHIBITION OF INSULIN AND GLUCAGON RELEASE INDUCED BY ARGININE *IN VIVO*.[172]

Peptide	Insulin	Glucagon	GH
SRIF	100	100	100
[Ala^2]-H_2SRIF	46	35	
[Ala^2]-SRIF	135	279	190
[D-Ala^2]-H_2SRIF			103
[D-Ala^2]-SRIF	227	240	55
[Ala^3]-H_2SRIF	< 10	< 10	< 0.1
[Ala^5]-H_2SRIF	112	176	
[Ala^5]-SRIF	132		130
[Ala^6]-H_2SRIF	< 10	< 10	
[Ala^6]-SRIF	< 10		1
[Ala^7]-H_2SRIF	< 10	< 10	
[Ala^7]-SRIF	< 10		3
[Ala^8]-H_2SRIF	< 10	< 10	
[Ala^8]-SRIF	< 10		< 0.5
[Ala^{10}]-H_2SRIF	< 10	< 10	
[Ala^{10}]-SRIF	14		25
[Ala^{11}]-H_2SRIF	29	< 10	
[Ala^{11}]-SRIF	< 10		2
[Ala^{12}]-H_2SRIF	22	< 10	
[Ala^{12}]-SRIF	26		4
[Ala^{13}]-H_2SRIF	< 10	< 10	
[Ala^{13}]-SRIF	27		6
[Ala^{14}]-H_2SRIF	< 10	< 10	0.5
[$Ala^{3,14}$]-H_2SRIF	< 10	< 10	0.6
[D-Trp^8]-H_2SRIF	123		89
[D-Trp^8]-SRIF	821	639	848

and (des-alanine^{1},glycine^{2}) histidine^{4,5},D-tryptophan^{8}-somatostatin have been reported to be more potent inhibitors of glucagon and growth hormone secretion than of insulin secretion.[167,169,171,173] The nonapeptides des-amino^{1,2,4,5,12}-D-tryptophan^{8},D-cysteine^{14}-somatostatin and des-amino^{1,2,4,5,13}-D-tryptophan^{8},phenylalanine^{12}-somatostatin have considerable selectivity and potency for glucagon.[224] Other analogues have been reported to be capable of inhibiting growth hormone but not insulin or glucagon secretion.[166,168] Several oligosomatostatin analogues such as des amino^{1,2,5,12,13}-D-tryptophan^{8}-somatostatin which do not possess increased intrinsic potency nevertheless have greatly enhanced durations of action (up to 18 hours); since this increased duration of action is observed when the compound administered subcutaneously but not intravenously, slow absorption from the injection site is the most likely explanation for this.[173]

The synthesis of potent analogues with significantly prolonged durations of action has recently been reported. WY40,973 has a 3-5 hour duration of action when given subcutaneously to diabetic dogs,[369] but also shows significant suppression of insulin secretion. Perhaps the most promising analogue developed to date is the des alanine^{1},glycine^{2} [His^{4,5}, D-Trp^{8}] somatostatin. This compound preferentially inhibits glucagon and growth hormone secretion; at appropriate doses, it can decrease circulating glucagon and growth hormone levels by 60 percent without affecting insulin levels. It is more potent than native somatostatin, and is active for up to 6-8 hours when given subcutaneously to dogs.[370] Bloom and associates, using several different analogues, have shown effective suppression of pancreatic endocrine tumors in man for up to 12 hours with a single subcutaneous dose.[371] More recently, conformational studies[372] suggesting a type II' β-turn from Phe[7] to Thr[10] and an antiparallel β-pleeted sheet structure involving Phe[6]- and Thr[10]-Phe[11] have led to the development of stable and long-acting somatostatin analogues which contain only 6-10 amino acids and are thus more readily synthesized in large quantities.[373]

It should be emphasized that most of the data regarding selective somatostatin analogues has been obtained either from *in vitro* studies or from studies in nonhuman species and, thus, whether these data are applicable to man is not yet known. Furthermore, the term selective has been used to indicate differences in the inhibition of insulin, glucagon, and growth hormone secretion. To date there is no evidence that any of the so-called selective analogues lack some of the other actions of somatostatin, e.g. its effects on the gastrointestinal tract.[364]

Remarkable progress has been made in the last five years toward the development of clinically useful somatostatin analogues. While formidable problems remain to be solved, it appears that a number of these agents will eventually be of value in the treatment of human disease. At present, efforts are underway to secure approval for the use of several analogues in clinical trials. Ultimately, it is likely that somatostatin analogues will play a role in the management of unresectable endocrine tumors of the pancreas, selected cases of acromegaly and perhaps most importantly, human diabetes mellitus.

ACKNOWLEDGEMENTS

The work reported herein from the author's laboratory was supported in part by grants from the USPHS (AM 20411, AM 20837, 074147, 05827), the Kroc Foundation and the Mayo Foundation. I am indebted to Ms. Cheryl Collins for her excellent editorial assistance.

REFERENCES

1. Burgus, R., Brazeau, P., and Vale, W., Isolation and determination of the primary structure of somatostatin (a somatotropin release inhibiting factor) of ovine hypothalamic origin, DHEW Publications, 1973, 74, (NIH) 144.

2. Vale, W., Brazeau, P., Rivier, C., Brown, M., Boss, B., Rivier, J., Bergus, R., Ling, N., and Guillemin, R., Somatostatin, Rec. Prog. Horm. Res., 34,365, 1975.

3. Burgus, R., Ling, N., Butcher, M., and Guillemin, R., Primary structure of somatostatin, a hypothalamic peptide that inhibits the secretion of pituitary growth hormone, Proc. Natl. Acad. Sci. USA, 79,684, 1973.

4. Schally, A., DuPont, A., Arimura, A., Redding, T., Nishi, N., Linthicum, G., and Schlessinger, D., Isolation and structure of somatostatin from porcine hypothalami, Biochemistry, 15,509, 1976.

5. Rivier, J., Somatostatin: Total solid phase synthesis, J. Am. Chem. Soc., 96,2986, 1974.

6. Arimura, A., Sato, H., DuPont, A., Nishi, N., and Schally, A., Somatostatin: Abundance of immunoreactive hormone in rat stomach and pancreas, Science, 189,1007, 1975.

7. Brownstein, M., Arimura, A., Sato, H., Schally, A., and Kizer, J., The regional distribution of somatostatin in the rat brain, Endocrinology, 96,1456, 1975.

8. Kronheim, S., Berelowitz, M., and Pimestone, B., A radioimmunoassay for growth hormone release-inhibiting hormone: Method and quantitative tissue distribution, Clin. Endocrinol., 5,619, 1976.

9. Patel, Y., and Reichlin, S., Somatostatin in hypothalamus, extrahypothalamic brain and peripheral tissues of the rat, Endocrinology, 102, 523, 1978.

10. Hokfelt, T., Efendic, S., Hellerstrom, C., Johansson, O., Luft, R., and Arimura, A., Cellular localization of somatostatin in endocrine-like cells and neurons of the rat with special references to the A_1-cells of the pancreatic islets and to the hypothalamus. Acta Endocrinol., 80 (Suppl. 200), 1, 1975.

11. Alpert, L., Brawer, J., Patel, Y., and Reichlin, S., Somatostatinergic neurons in anterior hypothalamus: Immunohistochemical localization. Endocrinology, 98,255, 1976.

12. Parsons, J., Erlandsen, S., Hegre, O., McEvoy, R., and Elde, R., Central and peripheral localization of somatostatin: Immunoenzyme immunohistochemical studies, J. Histochem. Cytochem., 24,872, 1976.

13. Hokfelt, T., Efendic, S., Johansson, O., Luft, R., and Arimura, A., Immunohistochemical localization of somatostatin (growth hormone release-inhibiting factor) in the guinea pig brain, Brain Res., 80, 165, 1974.

14. Desy, L., and Pelletier, G., Immunohistochemical localization of somatostatin in the human hypothalamus, Cell Tiss. Res., 184,491, 1977.

15. Bugnon, C., Fellmann, D., and Block, B., Immunocytochemical study of the ontogenesis of the hypothalamic somatostatin-containing neurons in the human fetus, Cell Tiss. Res., 183,319, 1977.

16. Pelletier, G., Labrie, F., Arimura, A., and Schally, A., Electron microscopic immunohistochemical localization of growth hormone release-inhibiting hormone (somatostatin) in the rat median eminence, Am. J. Anat., 140,445, 1974.

17. Pelletier, G., Dube, D., and Puviani, R., Somatostatin: Electron microscope immunohistochemical localization in secretory neurons of rat hypothalamus, Science, 196,1469, 1977.

18. Rufener, C., Amherdt, M., Dubois, M., and Orci, L., Ultrastructural immunocytochemical localization of somatostatin in rat pancreatic monolayer culture, J. Histochem. Cytochem., 24,866, 1976.

19. Rufener, C., Dubois, M., Mallaisse-Lagae, F., and Orci, L., Immunofluorescent reactivity to anti-somatostatin in the gastrointestinal mucosa of the dog, Diabetologia, 11,321, 1975.

20. Dubois, M., Immunoreactive somatostatin is present in discrete cells of the endocrine pancreas, Proc. Natl. Acad. Sci. USA, 72,1340, 1975.

21. Orci, L., Baetens, D., and Rufener, C., Evidence for the D-cell of the pancreas secreting somatostatin, Horm. Metab. Res., 7,400, 1975.

22. Goldsmith, P., Rose, J., Arimura, A., and Ganong, W., Ultrastructural localization of somatostatin in pancreatic islets of the rat, Endocrinology, 97,1061, 1975.

23. Polak, J., Grimelius, L., Pearse, A., Bloom, S., and Arimura, A., Growth-hormone release-inhibiting hormone in gastrointestinal and pancreatic D cells, Lancet, 1,1220, 1975.

24. Sundler, F., Aluments, J., Hakanson, R., Bjorklund, L., and Lundberg, O., Somatostatin-immunoreactive cells in medullary carcinoma of the thyroid, Am. J. Path., 88,381, 1977.

25. VanNoorden, S., Polak, J., and Pearse, A., Single cellular origin of somatostatin and calcitonin in the rat thyroid gland, Histochem., 53, 243, 1977.

26. Yamada, Y., Ito, S., Matsubara, Y., and Kobayashi, S., Immunohistochemical demonstration of somatostatin-containing cenns in the human, dog, and rat thyroids, Tohoku J. Exp. Med., 122,87, 1977.

27. Luft, R., Efendic, S., Hokfelt, T., Johansson, O., and Arimura, A., Immunohistochemical evidence for the localization of somatostatin-like immunoreactivity in a cell population of the pancreatic islets, Med. Biol., 52,428, 1974.

28. Pelletier, G., Identification of four cell types in the human endocrine pancreas by immunoelectron microscopy, Diabetes, 26,749, 1977.

29. Hokfelt, T., Elfvin, L., Elde, R., Schultzberg, M., Goldstein, M., and Luft, R., Occurrence of somatostatin-like immunoreactivity in some peripheral sympathetic noradrenergic neurons, Proc. Natl. Acad. Sci. USA, 74,3587, 1977.

30. Hokfelt, T., Johansson, O., Efendic, S., Luft, R., and Arimura, A., Are there somatostatin-containing nerves in the rat gut? Immunohistochemical evidence for a new type of peripheral nerves, Experientia, 31,852, 1975.

31. Patel, Y., Rao, K., and Reichlin, S., Somatostatin in human cerebrospinal fluid, New. Engl. J. Med., 296,529, 1977.

32. Kronheim, S., Berelowitz, M., and Pimestone, B., The presence of immunoreactive growth hormone release-inhibiting hormone in normal cerebrospinal fluid, Clin. Endocrinol., 6,411, 1977.

33. Kronheim, S., Berelowitz, M., and Pimestone, B., The characterization of growth hormone release inhibiting hormone-like immunoreactivity in normal urine, Clin. Endocrinol., 7,343, 1977.

34. Renaud, L., Martin, J., and Brazeau, P., Depressant action of TRH, LH-RH, and somatostatin on activity of central neurons, Nature, 255, 233, 1975.

35. Randic, M., and Miletic, V., Depressant actions of methionine-enkephalin and somatostatin in cat dorsal horn neurons activated by noxious stimuli, Brain Res., 152,196, 1978.

36. Tan, A., Tsang, D., Renaud, L., and Martin, J., Effect of somatostatin on calcium transport in guinea pig cortex synaptosomes, Brain Res. 123,193, 1977.

37. Havlicek, V., Rezek, M., and Friesen, H., Somatostatin and thyrotropin releasing hormone: Central effect on sleep and motor systems. Pharmacol. Biochem. Behav., 4,455, 1976.

38. Cohn, M., and Cohn, M., Barrel rotation induced by somatostatin in the non-lesioned rat, Brain Res., 96,138, 1975.

39. Brown, M., and Vale, W., Central nervous system effects of hypothalamic peptides, Endocrinology, 96,1333, 1975.

40. Koranyi, L., Whitmoyer, D., and Sawyer, C., Effect of thyrotropin-releasing hormone, luteinizing hormone-releasing hormone and somatostatin on neuronal activity of brain stem reticular formation and hippocampus in the female rat, Exptl. Neurol., 57,807, 1977.

41. Plotnikoff, N., Kastin, A., and Schally, A., Growth hormone release inhibiting hormone: Neuropharmacologic studies, Pharmacol. Biochem. Behav., 2,693, 1974.

42. Guillemin, R., Somatostatin inhibits the release of acetyl choline induced electrically in the myenteric plexus, Endocrinology, 99,1653, 1976.

43. Rezek, M., Havlicek, V., Hughes, K., and Friesen, H., Central site of action of somatostatin (SRIF): Role of hippocampus, Neuropharmacology, 15,499, 1976.

44. Cohen, M., Rosing, E., Wiley, K., and Slater, I., Somatostatin inhibits adrenergic and cholinergic neurotransmission in smooth muscle. Life Sci., 23,1659, 1978.

45. Gerich, J., Schultz, T., Tsalikian, E., Lorenzi, M., Lewis, S., and Karam, J., Clinical evaluation of somatostatin as a potential adjunct to insulin in the management of diabetes mellitus, Diabetologia, 13, 537, 1977.

46. Ashton, H., Millman, J., Telford, R., and Thompson, J., An electroencephalographic investigation of the short term effects of three hypothalamic hormones (TRH, LH/FSH-RH GH-RIH) in normal subjects, Br. J. Clin. Pharm., 3,523, 1976.

47. DuPont, E., Hansen, A., Juul-Jensen, P., Lundbaek, K., Magnussen, I., and DeFine Olivarius, B., Somatostatin in the treatment of patients with extrapyramidal disorders and patients with EEG abnormalities, Acta Neurol. Scand., 57,488, 1978.

48. Wakabayashi, I., Miyazawa, Y., Kanda, M., Miki, N., Demura, R., Demura, H., and Shizume, K., Stimulation of immunoreactive somatostatin release from hypothalamic synaptosomes by high (K^+) and dopamine, Endocrinol. Jap., 24,601, 1977.

49. Negro-Vilar, A., Ojeda, S., Arimura, A., and McCann, S., Dopamine and norepinephrine stimulate somatostatin release by median eminence fragments in vitro, Life Sci., 23,1493, 1978.

50. Patel, Y., Zingg, H., and Dreifuss, J., Calcium-dependent somatostatin secretion from rat neurohypophysis in vitro, Nature, 267,852, 1977.

51. Hall, R., Schally, A., Evered, D., Kastin, A., Mortimer, C., Turnbide, W., Besser, G., Coy, D., Goldie, D., McNeilly, A., Phenekos, C., and Weightman, D., Action of growth-hormone-release inhibitory hormone in healthy men and in acromegaly, Lancet, 2,581, 1973.

52. Besser, G., Mortimer, C., McNeilly, A., Thorner, M., Batistoni, G., Bloom, S., Kastrup, K., Hanssen, K., Hall, R., Coy, D., Kastin, A., and Schally, A., Long-term infusion of growth hormone release inhibiting hormone in acromegaly: Effects on pituitary and pancreatic hormones, Brit. Med. J., 4,622, 1974.

53. Besser, G., Mortimer, C., Carr, D., Schally, A., Coy, D., Evered, D., Kastin, A., Turnbridge, W., Thorner, M., and Hall, R., Growth hormone release inhibiting hormone in acromegaly, Br. Med. J., 1,352, 1974.

54. Peracchi, M., Reschini, E., Cantalamessa, L., Guistina, G., Cavagnini, F., Pinto, M., and Bulgheroni, P., Effect of somatostatin on blood glucose, plasma growth hormone, insulin, and free fatty acids in normal subjects and acromegalic patients, Metabolism, 23,1009, 1974.

55. Yen, S., Siler, T., and Devane, G., Effect of somatostatin in patients with acromegaly, New. Engl. J. Med., 290,935, 1974.

56. Pimestone, B., Becker, D., and Kronheim, S., Disappearance of plasma growth hormone in acromegaly and protein-calorie malnutrition after somatostatin, J. Clin. Endocrinol. Metab., 40,168, 1975.

57. Gerich, J., Lorenzi, M., Bier, D., Schneider, V., Tsalikian, E., Karam, J., and Forsham, P., Prevention of human diabetic ketoacidosis by somatostatin: Evidence for an essential role of glucagon, New Engl. J. Med., 292,985, 1975.

58. Christensen, S., Hansen, A., Weeke, J., and Lundbaek, K., 24-Hour studies of the effects of somatostatin on the levels of plasma growth hormone, glucagon, and glucose in normal subjects and juvenile diabetics, Diabetes, 27,300, 1978.

59. Laron, A., Pertzelan, A., Doron, M., Assa, S., and Keret, R., The effect of dihydrosomatostatin in dwarfism with high plasma immunoreactive growth hormone, Horm. Metab. Res., 9,338, 1977.

60. Raptis, S., Dollinger, H., Von Berger, L., Schlegel, W., Schroder, K., and Pfeiffer, E., Effects of somatostatin on gastric secretion and gastrin release in man, Digestion, 13,15, 1975.

61. Arimura, A., Smith, W., and Schally, A., Blockade of the stress-induced decrease in blood GH by anti-somatostatin serum in rats, Endocrinology, 98,540, 1976.

62. Ferland, L., Labrie, F., Jobin, M., Arimura, A., and Schally, A., Physiologic role of somatostatin in the control of growth hormone and thyrotropin secretion, Biochem. Biophys. Res. Commun., 68,149, 1976.

63. Terry, L., Willoughby, J., Brazeau, P., Martin, J., and Patel, Y., Antiserum to somatostatin prevents stress-induced inhibition of growth hormone secretion in the rat, Science, 192,565, 1976.

64. Tannenbaum, G., Epelbaum, J., Colle, E., Brazeau, P., and Martin, J., Antiserum to somatostatin reverses starvation-induced inhibition of growth hormone but not insulin secretion, Endocrinology, 102,1909, 1978.

65. Steiner, R., Stewart, J., Barber, J., Koerker, D., Goodner, C., Brown, A., Illner, P., and Gale, C., Somatostatin: A physiologic role in the regulation of growth hormone secretion in the adolescent male baboon, J. Clin. Endocrinol. Metab., 102,1587, 1978.

66. Baker, B., and Yen, Y., The influence of hypophysectomy on the stores of somatostatin in the hypothalamus and pituitary stem, Proc. Soc. Exptl. Biol. Med., 151,599, 1976.

67. Wakabayashi, I., Demura, R., Kanda, M., Demura, H., and Shizume, K., Effect of hypophysectomy on hypothalamic somatostatin content in rats, Endocrinol. Jap., 23,439, 1976.

68. Hoffman, D., and Baker, B., Effect of treatment with growth hormone on somatostatin in the median eminence of hypophysectomized rats, Proc. Soc. Exptl. Biol. Med., 156,265, 1977.

69. Fernandez-Durango, R. Arimura, A., Fishback, J., and Schally, A., Hypothalamic somatostatin and LH-RH after hypophysectomy, in hyper- or hypothyroidism and during anesthesia in rats, Proc. Soc. Exptl. Biol. Med., 157,235, 1978.

70. Weeke, J., Hansen, A., and Lundbaek, K., The inhibition by somatostatin of the thyrotropin response to thyrotropin-releasing hormone in normal subjects, Scand. J. Clin. Lab. Invest., 33,101, 1974.

71. Siler, T., Yen, S., Vale, W., and Guillemin, R., Inhibition by somatostatin of the release of TSH induced in man by thyrotropin-releasing factor, J. Clin. Endocrinol. Metab., 38,742, 1974.

72. Carr, D., Gomez-Pan, A., Weightman, D., Roy, V., Hall, R., Besser, G., Thorner, M., McNeilly, A., Schally, A., Kastin, A., and Coy, D., Growth hormone release inhibiting hormone: Actions on thyrotropin and prolactin secretion after thyrotropin-releasing hormone, Brit. Med. J., 3,67, 1975.

73. Weeke, J., Hansen, A., and Lundbaek, L., Inhibition by somatostatin of basal levels of serum thyrotropin (TSH) in normal man, J. Clin. Endocrinol. Metab., 41,168, 1975.

74. Lucke, C., Hoffken, B., and von zur Muhlen, A., The effect of somatostatin on TSH levels in patients with primary hypothyroidism, J. Clin. Endocrinol. Metab., 41,1082, 1975.

75. Florsheim, W., and Kozbur, X., Physiological modulation of thyrotropin secretion by somatostatin and thyroliberin, Biochem. Biophys. Res. Commun., 72,603, 1976.

76. Tanjasiri, P., Kozbur, X., and Florsheim, W., Somatostatin in the physiologic feedback control of thyrotropin secretion, Life Sci., 19, 657, 1976.

77. Chihara, K., Arimura, A., Chihara, M., and Schally, A., Studies on the mechanism of growth hormone and thyrotropin responses to somatostatin antiserum in anesthetized rats, Endocrinology, 103,1916, 1978.

78. Siler, T., Vandenberg, G., and Yen, S., Inhibition of growth hormone release in humans by somatostatin, J. Clin. Endocrinol. Metab., 37, 632, 1973.

79. Copinschi, G., Virasoro, E., Vanhaelst, L., Leclerq, R., Golstein, J., and L'Hermite, M., Specific inhibition by somatostatin of growth hormone release after hypoglycemia in normal man, Clin. Endocrinol., 3, 441, 1974.

80. Gerich, J., Davis, J., Lorenzi, M., Bohannon, N., Karam, J., Lewis, S., Kaplan, R., Schultz, T., and Cryer, P., Mechanisms of recovery from hypoglycemia in man. I. Interaction of glucagon and epinephrine, Am. J. Phys., 236,209, 1979.

81. Tyrrell J., Lorenzi, M., Gerich, J., and Forsham, P., Inhibition by somatostatin of ACTH secretion in Nelson's syndrome, J. Clin. Endocrinol. Metab., 40,1125, 1975.

82. Vale, W., Rivier, C., Brazeau, P., and Guillemin, R., Effects of somatostatin on the secretion of thyrotropin and prolactin, Endocrinology, 95,968, 1975.

83. Drovin, J., DeLean, A., Rainville, D., Lachance, R., and Labrie, F., Characteristics of the interaction between thyrotropin-releasing hormone and somatostatin for thyrotropin and prolactin release. Endocrinology, 98,514, 1976.

84. Benker, G., Hackenberg, K., Hamburger, B., and Reinwein, D., Effects of growth hormone release inhibiting hormone and bromocryptine (CB-154) in states of abnormal pituitary-adrenal function. Clin. Endocrinol, 5,187, 1976.

85. Fehr, H., Voigt, K., Lang, R., Beinert, K., Raptis, S., and Pfeiffer, E., Somatostatin: A potent inhibitor of ACTH-hypersecretion in adrenal insufficiency, Klin. Wschr., 54,173, 1976.

86. Deftos, L., Lorenzi, M., Bohannon, N., Tsalikian, E., Schneider, V., and Gerich, J., Somatostatin does not suppress plasma parathyroid hormone. J. Clin. Endocrinol. Metab., 43,205, 1976.

87. Gordin, A., Lamberg, B., Pelkonen, R., and Almquist, S., Somatostatin inhibits the pentagastrin-induced release of serum calcitonin in medullary carcinoma of the thyroid, Clin. Endocrinol., 8,289, 1978.

88. Ahren, B., Hedner, P., Melander, A., and Westgren, W., Inhibition by somatostatin of mouse thyroid activity following stimulation by thyrotropin, isoprenaline and dibutyryl cAMP, Acta Endocrinol., 86,323, 1977.

89. Loos, V., Raptis, S., Birk, J., Escobar-Jimenez, F., Maier, G., Voigt, K., Rothenbuchner, G., and Pfeiffer, E., Inhibition of TSH-mediated secretion of T_4, T_3, and reverse-T_3 in vivo and in isolated thyroid cells by somatostatin, Metabolism, 27(Suppl. 1),1269, 1978.

90. Faber, J., Gormsen, J., Frus, T., Kirkegaard, C., Lauridsen, V., Nerup, J., Rogowski, P., and Nielsen, K., Lack of effect of somatostatin on TSH induced T_3 release and platelet function in normal man, Horm. Metab. Res., 9,165, 1977.

91. Molnar, J., Arimura, A., and Kastin, A., Presence of somatostatin in the salivary gland and saliva, Fed. Proc., 35,782, 1976.

92. Forssman, W., Helmstaedter, V., Metz, J., Muhlmann, G., and Feurle, G., Immunohistochemistry and ultrastructure of somatostatin cells with special reference to the gastro-entero-pancreatic system, Metabolism, 27 (Suppl. 1),1179, 1978.

93. Falkmer, S., Elde, R., Hellerstrom, C., and Petersson, B., Phylogenetic aspects on somatostatin in the gastro-entero-pancreatic endocrine system, Metabolism, 27 (Suppl. 1),1193, 1978.

94. Helmstaedter, V., Feurle, G., and Forssman, W., Relationship of glucagon-somatostatin and gastrin-somatostatin cells in the stomach of the monkey, Cell Tiss. Res., 177,29, 1977.

95. McIntosh, C., Arnold, R., Bothe, E., Becker, H., Kobberling, J., and Creutzfeld, W., Gastrointestinal somatostatin in man and dog, Metabolism, 27 (Suppl. 1),1317, 1978.

96. vnas-Wallensten, K., Efendic, S., and Luft, R., Vagal release of somatostatin into the antral lumen of cats, Acta Physiol. Scand., 99, 126, 1977.

97. Uvnas-Wallensten, K., Lundberg, J., and Efendic, S., Dopaminergic control of antral gastrin and somatostatin release, Acta Physiol. Scand., 103,343, 1978.

98. Rizza, R., Miller, L., Go, V., and Gerich, J., Immunoreactive somatostatin-like material in human duodenal aspirates, Unpublished Observations.

99. Uvnas-Wallensten, K., Efendic, S., and Luft, R., Release of gastrointestinal hormones into the duodenal lumen of cats, Horm. Metab. Res., 10,173, 1978.

100. Uvnas-Wallensten, K., Efendic, S., and Luft, R., The occurrence of somatostatin-like immunoreactivity in the vagal nerves, Acta Physiol. Scand., 102,248, 1978.

101. Bloom, S., Mortimer, C., Thorner, M., Besser, G., Hall, R., Gomez-Pan, A., Roy, V., Russel, R., Coy, D., Kastin, A., and Schally, A., Inhibition of gastrin and gastric acid secretion by growth-hormone release-inhibiting hormone, Lancet, 2,1106, 1974.

102. Uvnas-Wallensten, K., Efendic, S., and Luft, R., Inhibition of vagally induced gastrin release by somatostatin in cats, Horm. Metab. Res., 9, 120, 1977.

103. Bolman, R., Cooper, C., and Wells, S., Somatostatin inhibition and reversal of parathyroid hormone-, calcium and acetylcholine-induced gastrin release in the pig, Endocrinology, 103,259, 1978.

104. Sclegel, W., Raptis, S., Dollinger, H., and Pfeiffer, E., Inhibition of secretin-, pancreozymin and gastrin release and their biological activities by somatostatin, in First International Symposium on Hormonal Receptors in Digestive Tract Physiology, Inserm Symposium No. 3, Bonfils, S., Fromageat, P., and Rosselin, G., Eds., Elsevier/North Holland Publishing Co., New York, 1977, 361.

105. Schrumpf, E., Vatn, M., Hanssen, K., Semb, L., and Myren, J., Somatostatin inhibits insulin-stimulated gastrin release and gastric secretion of acid, pepsin and intrinsic factor in duodenal ulcer patients, Scand. J. Gastroenterol., 11,517, 1976.

106. Creutzfeldt, W., and Arnold, R., Somatostatin and the stomach: Exocrine and endocrine aspects, Metabolism, 27 (Suppl. 1),1309, 1978.

107. Hayes, J., Johnson, D., Koerker, D., and Williams, R., Inhibition of gastrin release by somatostatin in vitro, Endocrinology, 96,1374, 1975.

108. Raptis, S., Dollinger, H., von Berger, L., Schlegel, W., Schroder, K., and Pfeiffer, E., Effects of somatostatin on gastric secretion and gastrin release in man, Digestion, 13,15, 1975.

109. Konturek, S., Tasler, J., Creszkowski, M., Coy, D., and Schally, V., Effect of growth-hormone release inhibiting hormone on gastric secretion, mucosal blood flow and serum gastrin, Gastroenterology, 70,737, 1976.

110. Raptis, S., Schlegel, W., Lehmann, E., Dollinger, H., and Zoupas, C., Effects of somatostatin on the exocrine pancreas and the release of duodenal hormones, Metabolism, 27 (Suppl.),1321, 1978.

111. Schlegel, W., Harvey, R., Raptis, S., Oliver, J., and Pfeiffer, E., inhibition of cholecystokinin-pancreozymin release by somatostatin, Lancet, 2,166, 1977.

112. Lennon, J., Sircus, W., Bloom, S., Mitchell, S., Polak, J., Besser, G., Hall, R., Coy, D., Kastin, A., and Schally, A., Investigation and treatment of a recurrent VIPoma, Gut, 16,821, 1975.

113. Sakurai, H., Dobbs, R., and Unger, R., The effect of somatostatin on the response of GLI to intraduodenal administration of glucose, protein and fat, Diabetologia, 11,427, 1975.

114. Bloom, S., Ralphs, D., Besser, G., Hall, R., Coy, D., Kastin, A., and Schally, A., Effect of somatostatin on motilin levels and gastric emptying, Gut, 16,834, 1975. (Abstract).

115. Pederson, R., Dryburgh, J., and Brown, J., The effect of somatostatin on release and insulinotropic action of gastric inhibitory polypeptide, Can. J. Physiol. Pharmacol., 53,1200, 1975.

116. Boden, G., Sivitz, M., Owen, O., Essa-Koumar, N., and Landor, J., Somatostatin suppresses secretin and pancreatic exocrine secretion, Science, 190,163, 1975.

117. Hanssen, L., Hanssen, K., and Myren, J., Inhibition of secretin release and pancreatic bicarbonate secretion by somatostatin in man. Scand. J. Gastroenterol., 12,391, 1977.

118. Marco, J., Hedo, J., and Villaneuva, M., Inhibitory effect of somatostatin on human pancreatic polypeptide secretion, Life Sci., 21,789, 1977.

119. Kayasseh, L., Haecki, W., Gyr, K., Stalder, G., Rittmann, W., Halter, F., and Girard, J., The endogenous release of pancreatic polypeptide by acid and meals in dogs: Effect of somatostatin, Scand. J. Gastroenterol., 13,385, 1978.

120. Barros, D'Sa, Bloom, S., and Baron, J., Direct inhibition of gastric acid by growth-hormone release-inhibiting hormone in dogs, Lancet, 1, 886, 1975.

121. Konturek, S., Radecki, T., Pucher, A., Coy, D., and Schally, A., Effect of somatostatin on gastrointestinal secretions and peptic ulcer formation in cats, Scand. J. Gastroenterol., 12,379, 1977.

122. Gomez-Pan, A., Albinus, M., Reed, J., Shaw, B., and Hall, R., Direct inhibition of gastric acid and pepsin secretion by growth-hormone release-inhibiting hormone in cats, Lancet, 1,88, 1975.

123. Schrumpf, E., Vatn, M., Hanssen, K., and Myren, J., A small dose of somatostatin inhibits the pentagastrin stimulated gastric secretion of acid, pepsin, and intrinsic factor in man, Clin. Endocrinol., 8,391, 1978.

124. Dollinger, H., Raptis, S., and Pfeiffer, E., Effects of somatostatin on exocrine and endocrine pancreatic function stimulated by intestinal hormones in man, Horm. Metab. Res., 8,74, 1976.

125. Wilson, R., Boden, G., Shore, L., and Essa-Koumar, N., Effect of somatostatin on meal-stimulated pancreatic exocrine secretions in dogs, Diabetes, 26,7, 1977.

126. Creutzfeldt, W., Lankisch, P., and Folsch, U., Hemmung der sekretin- und cholezystokinin-pancreozymin-induzierten saft-und enzymesekretion des pankreas und der gasllenblasenkontraktion beim menschen durch somatostatin, Dtsch. Med. Wschr., 100,1135, 1975.

127. Konturek, S., Tasler, J., Obtulowicz, W., Coy, D., and Schally, A., Effect of growth-hormone-release inhibiting hormone on hormones stimulating exocrine pancreatic secretion, J. Clin. Invest., 58,1, 1976.

128. Holm, I., Thulin, L., Samnegard, H., Efendic, S., and Tyden, G., Anticholeretic effect of somatostatin in anesthetized dogs, Acta Physiol. Scand., 104,241, 1978.

129. Tansy, M., Martin, J., Landin, W., and Kendall, F., The differential action of somatostatin on the motor effector system of the canine gastrointestinal tract, Metabolism, 27 (Suppl.),1353, 1978.

130. Thor, P., Krol, R., Konturek, S., Coy, D., and Schally, A., Effect of somatostatin on myoelectric activity of small bowel, Am. J. Physiol., 235,249, 1978.

131. Scholz, D., and Schwille, P., Somatostatin and intestinal calcium absorption in man, Metabolism, 27 (Suppl. 1),1349, 1978.

132. Krejs, G., Raskin, P., and Fordtran, J., Inhibition of jejunal sugar and amino acid absorption in man: A nonspecific effect of somatostatin, Clin. Res., 26,420A, 1978.

133. Carter, R., Bitar, K., Zfass, A., and Makhlouf, G., Inhibition of VIP-stimulated intestinal secretion and cyclic AMP production by somatostatin in the rat, Gastroenterology, 74,726, 1978.

134. Schwedes, U., Usadel, K., and Szabo, S., Somatostatin prevents cysteamine-induced duodenal ulcer, Eur. J. Pharmacol., 44,195, 1977.

135. Mattes, P., Raptis, S., Heil, T., Rasche, H., and Scheck, R., Extended somatostatin treatment of a patient with bleeding ulcer, Horm. Metab. Res., 7,508, 1975.

136. Lankisch, P., Koop, H., Winckler, K., Folsch, U., and Creutzfeldt, W., Somatostatin therapy of acute experimental pancreatitis, Gut, 18,713, 1977.

137. Reid, I., and Rose, J., An intrarenal effect of somatostatin on water excretion, Endocrinology, 100,782, 1977.

138. Brautbar, N., Levine, B., Coburn, J., and Kleeman, C., Interaction of somatostatin with PTH and AVP: renal effects, Am. J. Physiol., 237, 428, 1979.

138a. Le Roth, Bark, H., and Glick, S., Somatostatin and antidiuretic hormone secretion in dogs, Horm. Metab. Res., 11,177, 1979.

138b. Strandhoy, J., and Zook, T., Antagonism of vasopressin-induced water flow by somatostatin, Res. Commun. Chem. Path. Pharmacol., 24,599, 1979.

139. Gomez-Pan, A., Snow, M., Piercy, D., Robson, V., Wilkinson, R., Hall, R., Evered, C., Besser, G., Schally, A., Kastin, A., and Coy, D., Actions of growth hormone-release inhibiting hormone on the renin angiotensin system, J. Clin. Endocrinol. Metab., 43,240, 1976.

140. Rosenthal, J., Escobar-Jimenez, F., Raptis, S., and Pfeiffer, E., Inhibition of frusemide-induced hyperreninaemia by growth-hormone release-inhibiting hormone in man, Lancet, 1,772, 1976.

141. Rosenthal, J., Escobar-Jiminez, F., and Raptis, S., Prevention by somatostatin of rise in blood pressure and plasma renin mediated by beta-receptor stimulation, Clin. Endocrinol., 6,455, 1977.

142. Rosenthal, J., Raptis, S., Zoupas, C., and Escobar-Jiminez, F., Hemodynamic and renin responses to somatostatin in essential hypertension, Metabolism, 27 (Suppl. 1),1361, 1978.

143. Moulopoulos, S., Stamalelopoulos, S., and Vita, L., Somatostatin prolongation of the blood pressure lowering effect of diazoxide. Metabolism, 27 (Suppl. 1),1365, 1978.

144. Zierden, E., Hengst, K., and Wagner, H., Leukocyte response to somatostatin in normals and patients with bacterial leukocytosis. Klin. Wschr., 55,503, 1977.

145. Mielke, C., Gerich, J., Lorenzi, M., Tsalikian, E., Rodvien, R., and Forsham, P., The effect of somatostatin on coagulation and platelet function in man, New Engl. J. Med., 293,480, 1975.

146. Rasche, H., Raptis, S., Scheck, R., and Pfeiffer, E., Coagulation studies and platelet function after somatostatin, Klin. Wschr., 54, 977, 1976.

147. Bensoussan, D., Levy-Toledano, S., Passa, P., and Canivet, J., Effect of somatostatin on platelet aggregation and plasma factor. VIII level in normal man, Diabete et Metabolisme, 3,223, 1977.

148. Koerker, D., Harker, L., and Goodner, C., Effects of somatostatin on hemostasis in baboons, New Engl. J. Med., 293,476, 1975.

149. Zierden, E., Hengst, K., and Wagner, H., Influence of somatostatin on peripheral leukocyte count and granulation tissue in man and rats, Horm. Metab. Res., 9,378, 1977.

150. Chiang, T., Duckworth, W., Beachey, E., and Kang, A., The effect of somatostatin on platelet aggregation, Endocrinology, 97,753, 1975.

151. Besser, G., Paxton, A., Johnson, S., Moody, E., Mortimer, C., Hall, R., Gomez-Pan, A., Schally, A., Kastin, A., and Coy, D., Impairment of platelet function by growth-hormone release-inhibiting hormone, Lancet, 1,1166, 1975.

152. Mielke, C., and Rodvien, R., Somatostatin: Influence on hemostasis- a review, Metabolism, 27 (Suppl. 1),1369, 1978.

153. Scheck, R., Raptis, S., Rsche, H., and Escobar-Jiminez, F., The effect of somatostatin on platelets in vivo and in vitro studies. Diabete et Metabolisme, 3,219, 1977.

154. Guillemin, R., and Gerich, J., Somatostatin: Physiologic and clinical significance, Ann. Rev. Med., 27,379, 1976.

155. Luft, R., Efendic, S., and Hokfelt, T., Somatostatin-both hormone and neurotransmitter? Diabetologia, 14,1, 1978.

156. Pimestone, B., and Berelowitz, M., Somatostatin-paracrine and neuromodulator peptide in gut and nervous system, S. Afr. Med. J., 53,7, 1978.

157. Hansen, A., and Lundbaek, K., Somatostatin: A review of its effects especially in human beings, Diabete et Metabolisme, 2,203, 1976.

158. Lucke, C., Mitzkat, H., and von zur Muhlen, A., Somatostatin-a review, Klin. Wschr., 54,293, 1976.

159. Giustina, G., Peracchi, M., Reschini, E., Paneral, A., and Pinto, M., Dose-response study of the inhibiting effect of somatostatin on growth hormone and insulin secretion in normal subjects and acromegalic patients, Metabolism, 24,807, 1975.

160. Gerich, J., Lovinger, R., and Grodsky, G., Inhibition by somatostatin of glucagon and insulin release from the perfused rat pancreas in response to arginine, isoproterenol, and theophylline: Evidence for a preferential effect on glucagon secretion, Endocrinology, 96,749, 1975.

161. Bhathena, S., Perrino, P., Voyles, N., Smith, S., Wilkins, S., Coy, D., Schally, A., and Recant, L., Reversal of somatostatin inhibition of insulin and glucagon secretion, Diabetes, 25,1031, 1976.

162. Johnson, D., Ensinck, J., Koerker, D., Palmer, J., and Goodner, C., Inhibition of glucagon and insulin secretion by somatostatin in the rat pancreas perfused in situ, Endocrinology, 96,370, 1975.

163. Lorenzi, M., Karam, J., Schmitt, J., Burns, A., and Forsham, P., Hormonal, metabolic and gastrointestinal effects of low-and high dose somatostatin in man, Diabetes, 27, (Suppl. 2)442, 1978.

164. Coy, D., Meyers, C., Arimura, A., Schally, A., and Redding, T., Observations of the growth hormone, insulin, and glucagon release-inhibiting activities of somatostatin and analogues, Metabolism, 27 (Suppl. 1),1407, 1978.

165. Lien, E., and Garsky, V., Prolonged suppression of insulin release by a somatostatin analog, Endocrinology, 103,81, 1978.

166. Sarantakis, D., Teichman, J., Lien, E., and Fenichel, R., A novel cyclic undecapeptide, WY-40,770 with prolonged growth hormone release inhibiting activity, Biochem. Biophys. Res. Commun., 73,336, 1976.

167. Sarantakis, D., Teichman, J., Fenichel, R., and Lien, E., (des Ala^{1}, Gly^{2})-$His^{4,5}$, D-Trp^{8}-somatostatin, a glucagon-specific and long-acting somatostatin analog, FEBS Lett., 92,153, 1978.

168. Sarantakis, D., Teichman, J., Clark, D., and Grant, N., A bicyclo-somatostatin analog, highly specific for the inhibition of growth hormone release, Biochem. Biophys. Res. Commun., 75,143, 1977.

169. Meyers, C., Arimura, A., Gordin, A., Fernandez-Durango, R., Coy, D., Schally, A., Drouin, J., Ferland, L., Beaulieu, M., and Labrie, F., Somatostatin analogs which inhibit glucagon and growth hormone more than insulin release, Biochem. Biophys. Res. Commun., 74,630, 1977.

170. Efendic, S., Luft, R., and Sievertsson, H., Relative effects of somatostatin and two somatostatin analogues on the release of insulin, glucagon, and growth hormone, FEBS Lett., 58,302, 1975.

171. Efendic, S., Lins, P., Luft, R., Sievertsson, H., and Westin-Sjodal, G., Studies on the mechanism of somatostatin action on insulin release. V. Effect of somatostatin analogues on arginine induced release of insulin and glucagon from the perfused rat pancreas, Acta Endocrinol., 85,579, 1977.

172. Brown, M., Rivier, J., and Vale, W., Biologic activity of somatostatin and somatostatin analogues on inhibition of arginine-induced insulin and glucagon release in the rat, Endocrinology, 98,336, 1976.

173. Brown, M., Rivier, J., and Vale, W., Somatostatin analogs with selected biologic activities, Metabolism, 25 (Suppl. 1),1491, 1976.

174. Brown, M., Rivier, J., and Vale, W., Somatostatin: Analogs with selected biological activities, Science, 196,1467, 1977.

175. Fujimoto, W., Ensinck, J., and Williams, R., Somatostatin inhibits insulin and glucagon release by monolayer cell culture of rat endocrine pancreas, Life Sci., 15,1999, 1974.

176. Efendic, S., Luft, R., and Grill, V., Effect of somatostatin on glucose induced insulin release in isolated perfused rat pancreas and isolated rat pancreatic islets, FEBS Lett., 42,169, 1974.

177. Turcot-Lemay, L., Lemay, A., and Lacy, P., Somatostatin inhibition of insulin release from freshly isolated and organ cultured rat islets of Langerhans in vitro, Biochem. Biophys. Res. Commun., 63,1130, 1975.

178. Raptis, S., Escobar-Jiminez, F., Rosenthal, J., Ditschunet, H., and Pfeiffer, E., Somatostatin modulation of pancreatic glucagon, insulin, glucose and free fatty acids following beta-adrenergic stimulation, J. Clin. Endocrinol. Metab., 44,1088, 1977.

179. Curry, D., and Bennett, L., Does somatostatin inhibition of insulin secretion involve two mechanisms of action, Proc. Natl. Acad. Sci. USA, 73,248, 1976.

180. Curry, D., and Bennett, L., Direct inhibition of insulin secretion by synthetic somatostatin, Biochem. Biophys. Res. Commun., 58,885, 1974.

181. Fujimoto, W., Somatostatin inhibition of glucose-, tolbutamide-, theophylline, cytochalasin B-, and calcium-stimulated insulin release in monolayer cultures of rat endocrine pancreas, Endocrinology, 97, 1494, 1975.

182. Leblanc, H., and Yen, S., Comparison of cyclic and linear forms of somatostatin in the inhibition of growth hormone, insulin and glucagon secretion, J. Clin. Endocrinol. Metab., 40,906, 1975.

183. Leblanc, H., Anderson, J., Sigel, M., and Yen, S., Inhibitory action of somatostatin on pancreatic α and β cell function, J. Clin. Endocrinol. Metab., 40,568, 1975.

184. Alberti, K., Christensen, S., Iversen, J., Hansen, A., Christensen, N., Seyer-Hansen, K., Lundbaek, K., and Orskov, H., Inhibition of insulin secretion by somatostatin, Lancet, 2,1299, 1973.

185. Koerker, D., Ruch, W., Chideckel, E., Palmer, J., Goodner, C., Ensinck, J., and Gale, C., Somatostatin: Hypothalamic inhibitor of the endocrine pancreas, Science, 184,482, 1974.

186. Chideckel, E., Palmer, J., Koerker, D., Ensinck, J., Davidson, M., and Goodner, C., Somatostatin blockade of acute and chronic stimuli of the endocrine pancreas and the consequences of this blockade on glucose homeostasis, <u>J. Clin. Invest.</u>, 55,754, 1975.

187. Gerich, J., Lorenzi, M., Schneider, V., and Forsham, P., Effect of somatostatin on plasma gluccose and insulin responses to glucagon and tolbutamide in man, <u>J. Clin. Endocrinol. Metab.</u>, 39,1057, 1974.

188. Shapiro, S., Sumiya, E., Fleischer, N., and Baum, S., Regulation of in vitro insulin release from a transplantable Syrian hamster insulinoma, <u>Endocrinology</u>, 97,442, 1975.

189. Efendic, S., Luft, R., and Claro, A., Studies on the mechanism of somatostatin action on insulin release in man. II. Comparison of the effects of somatostatin on insulin release induced by glucose, glucagon, and tolbutamide, <u>Acta Endocrinol.</u>, 81,743, 1976.

190. Mortimer, C., Carr, D., Lind, T., Bloom, S., Mallinson, C., Schally, A., Turnbridge, W., Yeomans, L., Coy, D., Kastin, A., Besser, G., and Hall, R., Effects of growth-hormone release-inhibiting hormone on circulating glucagon, insulin, and growth hormone in normal, diabetic, acromegalic, and hypopituitary patients, <u>Lancet</u>, 1,697, 1974.

191. Efendic, S., Claro, A., and Luft, R., Studies on the mechanism of somatostatin action on insulin release. III. Effect of somatostatin on arginine induced release of insulin and glucagon in man and perfused rat pancreas, <u>Acta Endocrinol.</u>, 81,752, 1976.

192. Iversen, J., Inhibition of pancreatic glucagon release by somatostatin: in vitro, <u>Scand. J. Clin. Lab. Invest.</u>, 33,125, 1974.

193. Wollheim, C., Blondel, B., Renold, A., and Sharp, G., Somatostatin inhibition of pancreatic glucagon release from monolayer cultures and interactions with calcium, Endocrinology, 111,911, 1977.

194. Weir, G., Knowlton, S., and Martin, D., Somatostatin inhibition of epinephrine-induced glucagon secretion, Endocrinology, 95,1744, 1974.

195. Chideckel, E., Goodner, C., Koerker, D., Johnson, D., and Ensinck, J., Role of glucagon in mediating metabolic effects of epinephrine. Am. J. Physiol., 232,464, 1977.

196. Gerich, J., Lorenzi, M., Tsalikian, E., and Karam, J., Studies on the mechanism of epinephrine-induced hyperglycemia in man: Evidence for participation of pancreatic glucagon secretion, Diabetes, 25,65, 1976.

197. Gerich, J., Lorenzi, M., Karam, J., Schneider, V., and Forsham, P., Abnormal pancreatic glucagon secretion and postprandial hyperglycemia in diabetes mellitus, JAMA, 234,159, 1975.

198. Ward, F., Leblanc, H., and Yen, S., The inhibitory effect of somatostatin on growth hormone, insulin and glucagon secretion in diabetes mellitus, J. Clin. Endocrinol. Metab., 41,527, 1975.

199. Christensen, S., Hansen, A., and Lundbaek, K., Somatostatin in maturity-onset diabetes, Diabetes, 27,1013, 1978.

200. Christensen, S., Hansen, A., Weeke, J., and Lundbaek, K., 24 Hour studies of the effects of somatostatin on the levels of plasma growth hormone, glucagon, and glucose in normal subjects and juvenile diabetics, Diabetes, 27,300, 1978.

201. Griffey, M., Conway, H., Harshfield, D., and Whitney, J., Effect of somatostatin on insulin secretion induced by ionophore A23187, Proc. Soc. Exptl. Biol. Med., 154,198, 1977.

202. Taminato, T., Seino, Y., Goto, Y., and Imura, H., Interaction of somatostatin and calcium in regulating insulin release from isolated pancreatic islets of rats, Biochem. Biophys. Res. Commun., 66,928, 1975.

203. Taniguchi, H., Utsumi, M., Hasegawa, M., Kobayashi, T., Watanabe, Y., Murakami, K., Seki, M., Tsutou, A., Makimura, H., Sakoda, M., and Baba, S., Physiologic role of somatostatin: Insulin release from rat islets treated with somatostatin antiserum, Diabetes, 26,700, 1977.

204. Itoh, M., Mandarino, L., and Gerich, J., Antisomatostatin α-globulin augments secretion of both insulin and glucagon in vitro: evidence for a physiologic role for endogenous somatostatin in the regulation of pancreatic A and B cell function, Diabetes, 29, 1980, In Press.

205. Schusdziarra, V., Rouiller, D., Arimura, A., and Unger, R., Antisomatostatin serum increases levels of hormones from the pituitary and gut but not from the pancreas, Endocrinology, 103,1956, 1978.

206. Gerich, J., Lorenzi, M., Schneider, V., Kwan, C., Karam, J., Guillemin, R., and Forsham, P., Inhibition of pancreatic glucagon responses to arginine by somatostatin in normal man and in insulin-dependent diabetics, Diabetes, 23,876, 1974.

207. Christensen, N., Christensen, S., Hansen, A., and Lundbaek, K., The effect of somatostatin on plasma noradrenaline and plasma adrenaline concentrations during exercise and hypoglycemia, Metabolism, 24,1267, 1975.

208. Gerich, J., Lorenzi, M., Karam, J., Schneider, V., and Forsham, P., Abnormal pancreatic glucagon secretion and postprandial hyperglycemia in diabetes mellitus, JAMA, 234,159, 1975.

209. Wahren, J., and Felig, P., Influence of somatostatin in carbohydrate disposal and absorption in diabetes mellitus, Lancet, 2,1213, 1976.

210. Wagner, H., Hengst, K., Jansen, H., and Gerlach, V., Effects of somatostatin on absorption of mono- and disaccharides in small intestine in vivo and in vitro in man and rats, Metabolism, 27 (Suppl. 1), 1329, 1978.

211. Goldberg, D., Walesky, M., and Sherwin, R., Effect of somatostatin on the plasma amino acid response to ingested protein in man. Metabolism, In Press.

212. Liljenquist, J., Bloomgarden, Z., Cherrington, A., Perry, J., and Rabinowitz, D., Possible mechanism by which somatostatin-induced glucagon suppression improves glucose tolerance during insulinopenia in man, Diabetologia, In Press.

213. Cherrington, A., Chiasson, J., Liljenquist, J., Jennings, A., Keller, U., and Lacy, W., The role of insulin and glucagon in the regulation of basal glucose production in the postabsorptive dog, J. Clin. Invest., 58,1407, 1976.

214. Ishida, T., Rojdmark, S., Bloom, G., Chou, M., and Field, J., The effect of somatostatin on the hepatic extraction of insulin and glucagon in the anesthetized dog, Endocrinology, 104, 1979, In Press.

215. Sherwin, R., Tamborlane, W., Hendler, R., Sacca, L., DeFronzo, R., and Felig, P., Influence of glucagon replacement on the hyperglycemic and hyperketonemic response to prolonged somatostatin infusion in normal man, J. Clin. Endocrinol. Metab., 45,1104, 1977.

216. Altszuler, N., Gottlieb, B., and Hampshire, J., Interaction of somatostatin, glucagon, and insulin on hepatic glucose output in the normal dog, Diabetes, 25,116, 1976.

217. Alford, F., Bloom, S., Nabarro, J., Hall, R., Besser, G., Coy, D., Kastin, A., andd Scchally, A., Glucagon control of fasting glucose levels in man, Lancet, 2,974, 1974.

218. Blauth, C., Sonksen, P., Tompkins, C., and Bloom, S., The hypoglycemic action of somatostatin in the anesthetized dog, Clin. Endocrinol., 6,17, 1977.

219. Bryce, D., Yey, M., Funderburk, C., Todd, H., and Hertelendy, F., Studies on growth hormone secretion. VII. Effects of somatostatin on plasma GH, insulin and glucagon in sheep, Diabetes, 24,842, 1975.

220. Gerich, J., Lorenzi, M., Hane, S., Gustafson, G., Guillemin, R., and Forsham, P., Evidence for a physiologic role of pancreatic glucagon in human glucose homeostasis: Studies with somatostatin, Metabolism, 24,175, 1975.

221. Lins, P., and Efendic, S., Hyperglycemia induced by somatostatin in normal subjects, Horm. Metab. Res., 8,497, 1976.

222. Wahren, J., Efendic, S., Luft, R., Hagenfeldt, L., Bjorkman, O., and Felig, P., Influence of somatostatin on splanchnic glucose metabolism in postabsorptive and 60-hour fasted humans, J. Clin. Invest., 59,299, 1977.

223. Sherwin, R., Hendler, R., DeFronzo, R., Wahren, J., and Felig, P., Glucose homeostasis during prolonged suppression of insulin and glucagon by somatostatin, Proc. Natl. Acad. Sci. USA, 74,348, 1977.

224. Liljenquist, J., Mueller, G., Cherrington, A., Keller, V., Chiasson, J., Perry, J., Lacy, W., and Rabinowitz, D., Evidence for an important role of glucagon in the regulation of hepatic glucose production in normal man, J. Clin. Invest. 59,369, 1977.

225. Rizza, R., and Gerich, J., Does somatostatin cause sustained hyperglycemia in man? Clin. Res., 27,49A, 1979.

226. Gerich, J., Lorenzi, M., Schneider, V., Karam, J., Rivier, J., Guillemin, R., and Forsham, P., Effects of somatostatin on plasma glucose and glucagon levels in human diabetes mellitus: Pathophysiologic and therapeutic implications, New Engl. J. Med., 291,544, 1974.

227. Del Guercio, M., de Natale, G., Gargantini, L., Garlaschi, C., and Chiumello, G., Effect of somatostatin on blood sugar, plasma growth hormone, and glucagon levels in diabetic children, Diabetes, 25,550, 1976.

228. Gerich, J., Lorenzi, M., Bier, D., Tsalikian, E., Schneider, V., Karam, J., and Forsham, P., Effects of physiologic levels of glucagon and growth hormone on human carbohydrate and lipid metabolism: Studies involving administration of exogenous hormone during suppression of endogenous hormone secretion with somatostatn, J. Clin. Invest., 57,875, 1976.

229. Tamborlane, W., Sherwin, R., Hendler, R., and Felig, P., Metabolic effects of somatostatin in maturity-onset diabetes, New Engl. J. Med., 297,181, 1977.

230. Waldhausl, W., Bratusch-Marrain, P., Dudczak, R., and Deutsch, E., The diabetogenic action of somatostatin in healthy subjects and in maturity-onset diabetics, J. Clin. Endocrinol. Metab., 44,876, 1977.

231. Harano, Y., Ohgaku, S., Hidaka, H., Haneda, K., Kikawa, R., Shigeta, Y., And Abe, H., Glucose, insulin and somatostatin infusion for the determination of insulin sensitivity, J. Clin. Endocrinol. Metab., 45,1124, 1977.

232. Schusdziara, V., Brown, M., Rivier, J., Vale, W., Dobbs, R., Raskin, P., and Unger, R., Triglyceride lowering effect of somatostatin and its analogues, FEBS Lett., 79,133, 1977.

233. Raskin, P., and Unger, R., Hyperglucagonemia and its suppression: Importance in the metabolic control of diabetes, New Engl. J. Med., 299,433, 1978.

234. Tamborlane, W., Sherwin, R., Hendler, R., and Felig, P., Biphasic effect of somatostatin on oral glucose tolerance in maturity-onset diabetes, Metabolism, 27,849, 1978.

235. Meissner, C., Thum, C., Beischer, W., Winkler, G., Schroder, K., and Pfeiffer, E., Antidiabetic action of somatostatin--assessed by the artificial pancreas, Diabetes, 24,988, 1977.

236. Lundbaek, K., Hansen, A., Orskov, H., Christensen, S., Iversen, J., Seyer-Hansen, K., Alberti, K., and Whitefoot, R., Failure of somatostatin to correct diabetic ketoacidosis, Lancet, 1,214, 1976.

237. Christensen, S., Hansen, A., Orskov, H., and Lundbaek, K., 24-Hour somatostatin infusions in normals, juvenile diabetics, and maturity-onset diabetics, Metabolism, 27 (Suppl. 1),1427, 1978.

238. Jennings, A., Cherrington, A., Lilenquist, J., Keller, J., Lacy, W., and Chiasson, J., The roles of insulin and glucagon in the regulation of gluconeogenesis in the postabsorptive dog, Diabetes, 26,847, 1977.

239. Assan, R., Heuclin, C., Girard, J., Basdevant, A., Predine, J., and Husson, J., Hormonal and metabolic effects of somatostatin in diabetic patients submitted to an I.V. arginine infusion, Diabete et Metabolisme, 3,11, 1977.

240. Shulman, G., Liljenquist, J., Williams, P., Lacy, W., and Cherrington, A., Glucose disposal during insulinopenia in somatostatin-treated dogs, J. Clin. Invest., 62,487, 1978.

241. Sakurai, H., Dobbs, R., and Unger, R., Somatostatin-induced changes in insulin and glucagon secretion in normal and diabetic dogs, J. Clin. Invest., 54,1395, 1974.

242. Luyckx, A., and Lefebvre, P., Effect of somatostatin on metabolic and normal changes induced by nicotinic acid in insulin-dependent diabetics, Diabetologia, 12,447, 1976.

243. Lablanc, H., Rigg, L., and Yen, S., The response of pancreatic and pituitary hormones to pulses and constant infusion of somatostatin, J. Clin. Endocrinol. Metab., 41,1105, 1975.

244. Gerich, J., Schneider, V., Lorenzi, M., Tsalikian, E., Karam, J., Bier, D., and Forsham, P., Role of glucagon in human diabetic ketoacidosis studies with somatostatin, Clin. Endocrinol., 5, (Suppl) 299s, 1976.

245. Devane, G., Siler, T., and Yen, S., Acute suppression of insulin and glucose levels by synthetic somatostatin in normal human subjects, J. Clin. Endocrinol. Metab., 38,913, 1974.

246. Cherrington, A., Lacy, W., and Chiasson, J., Effect of glucagon on glucose production during insulin deficiency in the dog, J. Clin. Invest., 62,664, 1978.

247. Botha, J., Vinik, A., Roith, D., Child, P., and Jackson, W., The effects of somatostatin on hormonal and metabolic responses in chronic pancreatitis, S. Afr. Med. J., 51,872, 1977.

248. Bloomgarden, Z., Liljenquist, J., Cherrington, A., and Rabinowitz, D., Persistent stimulatory effect of glucagon on glucose production despite downregulation, J. Clin. Endocrinol. Metab., 47,1152, 1978.

249. Rizza, R., Verdonk, C., Miles, J., and Gerich, J., Effect of intermittent endogenous hyperglucagonemia on glucose homeostasis in normal and diabetic man, J. Clin. Invest., 63, 1979, In Press.

250. Curnow, R., Carey, R., Taylor, A., Johanson, A., and Murad, F., Somatostatin inhibitio of insulin and gastrin hypersecretion in pancreatic islet cell carcinoma, New Engl. J. Med., 292,1385, 1975.

251. Hirsch, H., Loo, S., Evans, N., Crigler, J., Filler, R., and Gabbay, K., Hypoglycemia of infancy and nesidioblastosis: Studies with somatostatin, New Engl. J. Med., 296,1323, 1977.

252. Locascio, V., Galvanini, G., Adami, S., Cinti, S., Bianchi, I., Cominacini, L., and Sairo, L., Failure of somatostatin to diagnose organic hyperinsulinism, Clin. Endocrinol., 8,81, 1978.

253. Lorenzi, M., Gerich, J., Karam, J., and Forsham, J., Failure of somatostatin to inhibit tolbutamide-induced insulin secretion in patients with insulinomas: A possible diagnostic tool, J. Clin. Endocrinol. Metab., 40,1121, 1975.

254. Scuro, L., Cascio, V., Adami, S., Galvani, G., Bianchi, I., Cominacini, L., and Corgnati, A., Somatostatin inhibition of insulin secretion in insulin-producing tumors, Metabolism, 25,603, 1976.

255. Tiengo, A., Fedele, D., Marchiori, E., Nosadini, R., and Muggeo, M., Suppression and stimulation mechanisms controlling glucagon secretion in a case of islet-cell tumors producing glucagon, insulin, and gastrin, Diabetes, 25,408, 1976.

256. Hertelendy, F., Calabria, D., Todd, H., and Raab, B., Somatostatin inhibits urinary cyclic AMP excretion in diabetic rats, Endocrinology, 101,1095, 1977.

257. Herchl, R., Havlicek, V., Rezek, M., and Kroeger, E., Cerebroventricular administration of somatostatin: Effect on central levels of cyclic AMP, Life Sci., 20,821, 1977.

258. Dobbs, R., Sakurai, H., Sasaki, H., Faloona, G., Valverde, I., Baetens, D., Orci, L., and Unger, R., Glucagon: Role in the hyperglycemia of diabetes mellitus, Science, 187,544, 1975.

259. Christensen, S., Hansen, A., Iversen, J., Lundbaek, K., Orskov, H., and Seyer-Hansen, K., Somatostatin as a tool in studies of basal carbohydrate and lipid metabolism in man: Modifications of glucagon and insulin release, Scand. J. Clin. Lab. Invest., 34,321, 1974.

260. Copinschi, G., Leclercq-Meyer, V., Virasoro, E., L'Hermite, M., Vanhaelst, L., Golstein, J., Leclercq, R., Fery, F., and Robyn, C., Pituitary and extrapituitary effects of somatostatin in normal man, Horm. Metab. Res., 8,226, 1976.

261. Johnston, D., Gill, A., Hanson, R., Alberti, K., Batstona, and Orskov, H., Somatostatin: A tool for investigation of the metabolic effects of cortisol and glucagon, Metabolism, 27 (Suppl. 1),1445, 1978.

262. Cherrington, A., Caldwell, M., Dietz, M., Exton, J., and Crofford, O., The effect of somatostatin on glucose uptake and production by rat tissues in vitro, Diabetes, 26,740, 1977.

263. Byrne, R., Nompleggi, D., Ramey, E., and Penhos, J., Studies on the extrapancreatic metabolic effects of somatostatin, Proc. Soc. Exptl. Biol. Med., 155,507, 1977.

264. Verdonk, C., Rizza, R., and Gerich, J., Effect of somatostatin-induced glucagon deficiency on fasting plasma glucose levels and glucose turnover rates in normal man, Unpublished Observations.

265. Olsson, S., Andersson, A., Petersson, B., and Hellerstrom, C., Effects of somatostatin on the biosynthesis and release of insulin from isolated pancreatic islets, Diabete et Metabolisme, 2,199, 1976.

266. Lin, B., Effects of somatostatin on insulin biosynthesis, glucose oxidation and cyclic guanosine monophosphate level, Metabolism, 27 (Suppl. 1),1295, 1978.

267. Schonbrunn, A., and Tashjian, A., Characterization of functional receptors for somatostatin in rat pituitary cells in culture, J. Biol. Chem., 253,6473, 1978.

268. Rifkin, R., Leitner, J., Maman, A., and Sussman, K., Localization of somatostatin binding in somatostatin responsive tissues, Clin. Res., 27,87A, 1979.

269. Rizza, R., and Gerich, J., Somatostatin receptors in pancreatic islet plasma membrane, Unpublished Observations.

270. Pace, C., Murphy, M., Conant, S., and Lacy, P., Somatostatin inhibition of glucose-induced electrical activity in cultured rat islet cells, Am. J. Physiol., 233,C164, 1977.

271. Ogawa, H., Thompson, T., Friesen, H., Martin, J., and Brazeau, P., Properties of soluble somatostatin-binding protein, Biochem. J., 165, 269, 1977.

272. Sussman, K., Keitner, J., and Rifkin, R., Somatostatin: Selective inhibition of cyclic AMP stimulated protein kinase activity in isolated pancreatic islet and pituitary secretory vesicles, Clin. Res., 26, 563A, 1978.

273. Rasmussen, H., and Goodman, D., Relationship between calcium and cyclic nucleotides in cell activation, Physiol. Rev., 57,421, 1977.

274. Malaisse, W., Calcium ion fluxes and insulin release in pancreatic islets, Biochem. Soc. Trans., 5,872, 1977.

275. Grodsky, G., A threshold distribution hypothesis for packet storage of insulin. II. Effect of calcium, Diabetes, 21, (Suppl. 2)584, 1972.

276. Curry, D., and Bennett, L., Reversal of somatostatin inhibition of insulin secretion by calcium, Biochem. Biophys. Res. Commun., 60, 1015, 1974.

277. Basabe, J., Cresto, J., and Aparicio, N., Studies on the mode of action of somatostatin on insulin secretion, Endocrinology, 101,1436, 1977.

278. Fujimoto, W., and Ensinck, J., Somatostatin inhibition of insulin and glucagon secretion in rat islet culture. Reversal by ionophore A23187, Endocrinology, 98,259, 1976.

279. Oliver, J., Inhibition of calcium uptake by somatostatin in isolated rat islets of Langerhans, Endocrinology, 99,910, 1976.

280. Schofield, J., and Bicknell, R., Effects of somatostatin and verapamil on growth hormone release and ^{45}Ca fluxes, Molec. Cell Endocrinol., 9,255, 1978.

281. Shapiro, S., Kaneko, Y., Baum, S., and Fleischer, N., The role of calcium in insulin release from hamster insulinoma cells, Endocrinology, 101,485, 1977.

282. Wollheim, C., Kikuchi, M., Renold, A., and Sharp, G., Somatostatin- and epinephrine-induced modifications of $^{45}Ca^{++}$ fluxes and insulin release in rat pancreatic islets maintained in tissue culture, J. Clin. Invest., 60,1165, 1977.

282a. Bicknell, R., and Schofield, J., Mechanism of action of somatostatin: Inhibition of ionophore A23187-induced release of growth hormone from dispersed bovine pituitary cells, FEBS Lett., 68,23, 1976.

283. Mandarino, L., Itoh, M., Blanchard, W., Patton, G., and Gerich, J., Stimulation of insulin release in the absence of extracellular calcium by isobutylmethylxanthine and its inhibition by somatostatin, Endocrinology, 106, 1980, In Press.

284. Borgeat, P., Labrie, P., Crouin, J., Belanger, A., Immer, H., Sestanj, K., Ivelson, V., Gotz, M., Schally, A., Coy, D., and Coy, E., Inhibition of adenosine 3',5' monophosphate accumulation in anterior pituitary gland in vitro by growth hormone release inhibiting hormone, Biochem. Biophys. Res. Commun., 56,1052, 1974.

285. Kaneko, T., Oka, H., Munemura, M., Suzuki, S., Yasuda, H., Oda, T., and Yanaihara, N., Stimulation of guanosine 3',5' cyclic monophosphate accumulation in rat anterior pituitary gland in vitro by synthetic somatostatin, Biochem. Biophys. Res. Commun., 61,53, 1974.

286. Efendic, S., Grill, V., and Luft, R., Inhibition by somatostatin of glucose induced 3',5'-monophosphate (cyclic AMP) accumulation and insulin release in isolated pancreatic islets of the rat, FEBS Lett., 55,131, 1975.

287. Oliver, J., and Wagle, S., Studies on the inhibition of insulin release, glycogenolysis, and gluconeogenesis by somatostatin in the rat islets of Langerhans and isolated hepatocytes, Biochem. Biophys. Res. Commun., 62,772, 1975.

288. Oliver, J., Wright, P., and Ashmore, J., The effect of somatostatin on glucose stimulated adenosine 3',5' monophosphate accumulation and glucose oxidation by isolated rat islets of Langerhans, Proc. Soc. Exptl. Biol. Med., 158,458, 1978.

289. Bicknell, R., Young, P., and Schofield, J., Mechanism of action of somatostatin: Growth hormone release ^{45}Ca ion efflux and cyclic nucleotide metabolism of bovine anterior pituitary slices in the presence of prostaglandin E_2 and 1-methyl-e-isobutylxanthine, Proc. Biochem. Soc., 5,219, 1977.

290. Charles, M., Larvecki, J., Steiner, A., and Grodsky, G., Cyclic nucleotides in pancreatic islets: Tolbutamide and arginine-induced insulin release, Diabetes, 25,256, 1976.

291. Claro, A., Grill, V., Efendic, S., and Luft, R., Studies on the mechanisms of somatostatin action on insulin release. IV. Effect of somatostatin on cyclic AMP levels and phosphodiesterase activity in isolated rat pancreatic islets, Acta Endocrinol., 85,379, 1977.

292. Kemmler, W., and Loffler, G., NaK-ATPase in rat pancreatic islets, Diabetologia, 13,235, 1977.

293. Smith, P., Woods, S., Ensinck, J., and Porte, D., Phentolamine prevents the somatostatin-mediated inhibition of pancreatic glucagon secretion, Metabolism, 26,841, 1977.

294. Smith, P., Woods, S., and Porte, D., Phentolamine blocks the somatostatin-mediated inhibition of insulin secretion, Endocrinology, 98, 1073, 1976.

295. Schmitt, J., Lorenzi, M., Gerich, J., Bohannon, N., Karam, J., and Forsham, P., Effect of phentolamine on somatostatin's action in man, Clin. Res., 26,131A, 1978.

296. Efendic, S., and Luft, R., Studies on the mechanism of somatostatin action on insulin release in man. I. Effect of blockade on α-adrenergic receptors, Acta Endocrinol., (K6H) 78,516, 1975.

297. Kaneto, A., Kajinuma, H., Kaneto, T., and Kosaka, K., Effect of phentolamine on the somatostatin-induced inhibition of glucagon and insulin secretion, Metabolism, 27,901, 1978.

298. Hara, M., Patton, G., and Gerich, M., Effect of alpha adrenergic blockade on inhibition by somatostatin of insulin release from the in vitro perfused rat pancreas. Program 60th Annual Meeting of the Endocrine Society, June 14-16, Miami Beach, 1978, 466.

299. Schusdziarra, V., Harris, V., and Unger, R., Half-life of somatostat-in-like immunoreactivity in canine plasma, Endocrinology, 104,109, 1979.

300. Sheppard, M., Shapiro, B., Berelowitz, M., and Pimestone, B., Metabolic clearance and plasma half disappearance time of exogenous somatostatin in man, J. Clin. Endocrinol. Metab., 48,50, 1979.

301. Ensinck, J., Laschansky, E., Chideckel, E., Palmer, J., and Goodner, C., Somatostatin kinetic during infusion in the baboon, Clin. Res., 24,155A, 1976.

302. Shapiro, B., Sheppard, M., Kronheim, S., and Pimestone, B., Transrenal gradient of serum somatostatin-like immunoreactivity in the rat, Horm. Metab. Res., 10,356, 1978.

303. Marks, N., and Stern, F., Inactivation of somatostatin (GH-RIH) and its analogues by crude and partially purified rat brain extracts, FEBS Lett., 55,220, 1975.

304. Griffiths, E., Jeffcoate, S., and Holland, D., Inactivation of somatostatin by peptidases in different areas of the rat brain, Acta Endocrinol., 85,1, 1977.

305. Marks, N., Stern, F., and Benuck, M., Correlation between biologic potency and biodegradation of a somatostatin analogue, Nature, 261, 511, 1976.

306. Patton, G., Rizza, R., and Gerich, J., Degradation of synthetic somatostatin by isolated guinea pig pancreatic acinar cells and by the perfused rat pancreas, Unpublished Observations.

307. Benuck, M., and Marks, N., Differences in the degradation of hypothalamic releasing factors by rat and human serum, Life Sci., 19, 1271, 1976.

308. Dupont, A., Merand, Y., and Barden, N., Effect of propylthiouracil and thyroxine on the inactivation of somatostatin by rat hypothalamus, Life Sci., 23,2007, 1978.

309. Berelowitz, M., Pimestone, B., Shapiro, B., Kronheim, S., and DeWitt, D., Tissue growth hormone release inhibiting hormone-like immunoreactivity in experimental hypothyroidism and hypopituitarism, Clin. Endocrinol., 9,185, 1978.

310. Barden, N., Alvarado-Urbina, G., Cote, J., and Dupont, A., Cyclic AMP-dependent stimulation of somatostatin secretion by isolated rat islets of Langerhans, Biochem. Biophys. Res. Commun., 71,840, 1976.

311. Schauder, P., McIntosh, C., Arends, J., Arnold, R., Ferichs, H., and Creutzfeldt, W., Somatostatin and insulin release from isolated rat pancreatic islets stimulated by glucose, FEBS Lett., 68,225, 1976.

312. Patton, G., Ipp, E., Dobbs, R., Orci, L., Vale, W., and Unger, R., Response of pancreatic immunoreactive somatostatin to arginine, Life Sci., 19,1957, 1976.

313. Patton, G., Ipp, E., Dobbs, R., Orci, L., Vale, W., and Unter, R., Pancreatic immunoreactive somatostatin release, Proc. Natl. Acad. Sci. USA, 74,2140, 1977.

314. Schauder, P., McIntosh, C., Paten, U., Arends, J., Frerichs, H., and Creutzfeldt, W., Dynamics of somatostatin release from isolated rat pancreatic islets, FEBS Lett., 81,355, 1977.

315. Ipp, E., Dobbs, R., Arimura, A., Vale, W., Harris, V., and Unger, R., Release of immunoreactive somatostatin from the pancreas in response to glucose, amino acids, pancreozymin-cholecystokinin, and tolbutamide, J. Clin. Invest., 60,760, 1977.

316. Schauder, P., McIntosh, C., Arends, J., Arnold, R., Frerichs, H., and Creutzfeldt, W., Somatostatin and insulin release from isolated rat pancreatic islets in resonse to D-glucose, L-leucine, α-ketoisocaproic acid or D-glyceraldehyde: evidence for a regulatory role of adenosine-3',5' cyclic monophosphate, Biochem. Biophys. Res. Commun., 75,630, 1977.

317. Ipp, E., Dobbs, R., Harris, V., Arimura, A., Vale, W., and Unger, R., The effects of gastrin, gastric inhibitory polypeptide, secretin, and the actapeptide of cholecystokinin upon immunoreactive somatostatin release by the perfused canine pancreas, J. Clin. Invest., 60,1216, 1977.

318. Efendic, S., Nylen, A., Roovete, A., and Uvnas-Wallenstein, K., Effects of glucose and arginine on the release of immunoreactive somatostatin from the isolated perfused rat pancreas, FEBS Lett., 92, 33, 1978.

319. Ipp, E., Dobbs, R., and Unter, R., Vasoactive intestinal peptide stimulates pancreatic somatostatin release, FEBS Lett., 90,76, 1978.

320. Ipp, E., Dobbs, R., and Unger, R., Morphine and β-endorphin influence the secretion of the endocrine pancreas, Nature, 276:190, 1978.

321. Barden, N., Cote, J., Lavoie, M., and Dupont, A., Secretion of somatostatin by rat islets of Langerhans and gastric mucosa and a role for pancreatic somatostatin in the regulation of glucagon release, Metabolism, 27 (Suppl. 1),1215, 1978.

322. Gerich, J., Greene, K., Hara, M., Rizza, R., and Patton, G., Radioimmunoassay of somatostatin and its application in the study of pancreatic somatostatin secretion in vitro, J. Lab. Clin. Med., 93,1009, 1979.

323. Hara, M., Patton, G., and Gerich, J., Increased release of somatostatin from pancreases of alloxan diabetic rats perfused in vitro, Life Sci., 24,625, 1979.

324. Weir, G., Samols, E., Loo, S., Patel, Y., and Gabbay, K., Somatostatin and pancreatic polypeptide secretion: effects of glucagon, insulin, and arginine, Diabetes, 28,35, 1979.

325. Schauder, R., McIntosh, C., Arends, J., and Frerichs, H., Effect of fasting on the release of insulin and somatostatin from perfused islets of Langerhans, Diabetes, 28,204, 1979.

326. Samols, E., and Weir, G., Adrenergic modulation of pancreatic A, B, and D cells: α-adrenergic suppression of β-adrenergic stimulation of somatostatin secretion, α-adrenergic stimulation of glucagon secretion in the perfused dog pancreas, J. Clin. Invest., 63,230, 1979.

327. Ipp, E., Rivier, J., Dobbs, R., Brown, J., Vale, W., and Unger, R., Somatostatin analogs inhibit somatostatin release, Endocrinology, 104,1270, 1979.

328. Petersson, B., Lundquist, G., and Anderson, A., Somatostatin content and release of isolated pancreatic islets from obese-hyperglycemic ice, Experientia, 35,127, 1979.

329. Patel, Y., Amherdet, M., and Orci, L., Somatostatin secretion from monolayer cultures of neonatal rat pancreas, Endocrinology, 104,676, 1979.

330. Honey, R., and Weir, G., Insulin stimulates somatostatin and inhibits glucagon secretion from the perfused chicken pancreas-duodenum. Life Sci., 24,1747, 1979.

331. Barden, N., Dube, D., Cote, J., Leclercq, R., and Pelletier, G., Immunohistochemical characterization of monolayer cell cultures of embryonic chicken pancreas and measurements of somatostatin release, J. Histochem. Cytochem., 27,939, 1979.

332. Dolais-Kitabgi, J., Kitabgi, P., Brazeau, P., and Freychet, P., Effect of neurotensin on insulin, glucagon, and somatostatin release from isolated pancreatic islets, Endocrinology, 105,256, 1979.

333. Goto, Y., Seino, Y., Taminato, T., Kadowaki, S., Chiba, T., Note, S., and Imura, H., Theophylline: protentiation of arginine-induced somatostatin release from the isolated rat pancreas, Diabetes, 28,457, 1979.

334. Hermansen, K., Christensen, S., and Orskov, H., Characterization of somatostatin release from the pancreas: the role of calcium and acetylcholine, Diabetologia, 16,261, 1979.

335. Kadowaki, S., Taminato, Taminato, T., Chiba, T., Mori, K., Abe, H., Goto, Y., Seino, Y., Matsukura, S., Nozawa, M., and Fujita, T., Somatostatin release from isolated perfused rat pancreas: possible role of endogenous somatostatin on insulin release, Diabetes, 28,600, 1979.

336. Lee, S., Havlicek, V., Panerai, A., and Friesen, H., High K^+-induced release of somatostatin from the cortical preparation of rat brain, Experientia, 35,351, 1979.

337. Patel, Y., Zingg, H., and Dreifuss, J., Calcium-dependent somatostatin secretion from rat neurohypophysis in vitro, Nature, 267,852, 1977.

338. Iversen, L., Iversen, S., Bloom, F., Douglas, C., Brown, M., and Vale, W., Calcium-dependent release of somatostatin from rat brain in vitro, Nature, 273,161, 1978.

339. Bennett, G., Edwardson, J., DeCotte, D., Berelowitz, M., Kronheim, S., Pimestone, B., and Sheppard, M., Potassium stimulated calcium dependent release of immunoreactive somatostatin from incubated rat hypothalamus, J. Neurochem., 31,1537, 1978.

340. Wakabayashi, I., Miyazawa, Y., Kanda, M., Miki, N., Demura, R., Demura, H., and Shizume, K., Stimulation of immunoreactive somatostatin release from hypothalamic synaptosomes by high (K^+) and dopamine, Endocrinol. Jap., 24,601, 1977.

341. Negro-Vilar, A., Ojeda, S., Arimura, A., and McCann, S., Dopamine and norepinephrine stimulate somatostatin release by median eminence fragments in vitro, Life Sci., 23,1493, 1978.

342. Uvnas-Wallensten, K., Efendic, S., and Luft, R., Vagal release of somatostatin into the antral lumen of cats, Acta Physiol. Scand., 99, 126, 1977.

343. Uvnas-Wallensten, K., Lundberg, J., and Efendic, S., Dopaminergic control of antral gastrin and somatostatin release, Acta Physiol. Scand., 103,343, 1978.

344. Chihara, K., Arimura, A., and Schally, A., Effect of intraventricular injection of dopamine, norepinephrine, acetylcholine, and 5-hydroxytryptamine on immunoreactive somatostatin release into rat hypophysical portal blood, Endocrinology, 104,1656, 1979.

345. Creutzfeldt, W., Zur deutung des silberzellbildes und anderer pankreasbefunde beim diabetes mellitus und inseladonom, Beitrog. Pathol. Anat., 113,133, 1953.

346. Gepts, W., Die histopathologischen veranderungen des longerhansschen inselin und irher bedeutung in der frage der pathogenese des menschlichen diabetes, Endokrinologie, 36,185, 1958.

347. Ferner, H., Beitrage zur histologic der longerhaneschen inseln des menchen mit besonderer berucksichtung der silberzellen und ihrer beziehung zum pankreasdiabetes, Virchows Arch. Pathol. Anat., 309, 136, 1942.

348. Fujita, T., D-zellern der pankreasinseln beim diabetes mellitus met besonderer beruchsichtunp ihrer argyrophibe, Z. Zellforsch, 69,363, 1976.

349. Hellman, B., and Petersson, B., Longterm changes of the A_1 and A_2 cells in the islets of rats with alloxan diabetes, Endocrinology, 72,238, 1963.

350. Kobayaski, K., Takahashi, Y., and Yohshita, T., Influences of alloxan administration and hypophysectomy on the pancreatic islets of the rat, Arch. Histol. Japon., 25,199, 1964.

351. Stefan, Y., Malaisse-Lagae, F., Yoon, J., Notkins, A., and Orci, L., Virus-induced diabetes in mice: A quantitative evaluation of islet cell population by immunofluoresence technique, Diabetologia, 15,395, 1978.

352. Petersson, B., Elde, R., Efendic, S., Hokfelt, T., Johansson, O., Lufh, R., Cerasi, E., and Hellerstrom, C., Somatostatin in the pancreas, stomach, and hypothalamus of the diabetic chinese hamster, Diabetologia, 13,463, 1977.

353. Baetens, D., Stefan, Y., Ravazzola, M., Malaisse-Lagae, F., Coleman, D., and Orci, L., Alteration of islet cell populations in spontaneously diabetic mice, Diabetes, 27,1, 1978.

354. Matsushima, Y., Makino, H., Kanatsuka, A., Yamamoto, M., and Kumagi, A., Immunohistochemical changes of somatostatin cells in the pancreatic islets of rats after streptozotocin administration, Endocrinol. Japon., 25,111, 1978.

355. Jaspen, J., Polonsky, K., Lewis, M., and Moosa, A., Reduction in portal vein blood flow by somatostatin, Diabetes, 28,888, 1979.

356. Tyden, G., Somnegard, H., Thulen, L., and Freman, L., Treatment of bleeding esophageal varices with somatostatin, N. Engl. J. Med., 299, 1466, 1978.

357. Schusdziarra, V., Rivier, J., Dobbs, R., Brown, M., Vale, W., and Unter, R., Somatostatin analogues as glucagon suppressants in diabetes, Horm. Metab. Res., 10,563, 1978.

358. Turchiana, M., Stone, C., Cook, P., and Weise, S., Effect of new synthetic analogs of somatostatin on gastric secretion in the chronic fistula dog, Proc. Soc. Exptl. Biol. Med., 154,449, 1977.

359. Sarantakis, D., McKinley, W., and Grant, N., The synthesis and biologic activity of $Ala^{3,14}$-somatostatin, Biochem. Biophys. Res. Commun., 55,538, 1973.

360. Rivier, J., Brazeau, P., Vale, W., and Guillemin, R., Somatostatin analogues: Relative imortance of the disulfide bridge and of the Ala-Gly side chain for biologic activity, J. Med. Chem., 18,123, 1975.

361. Rivier, J., Brown, M., and Vale, W., Tyrosylated analogs of somatostatin, J. Med. Chem., 19,1010, 1976.

362. Rivier, J., Brown, M., and Vale, W., D-Trp^{8}-somatostatin: An analogue of somatostatin more potent than the native molecule, Biochem. Biophys. Res. Commun., 65,746, 1975.

363. Lien, E., Fenichel, R., Grant, N., Boxill, G., Greenwood, J., and Yardley, J., Prolonged suppression of pituitary and pancreatic hormone release by a somatostatin analog, Biochem. Biophys. Res. Commun., 77,1317, 1977.

364. Konturek, S., Tasler, J., Krol, R., Dembinski, A., Coy, D., and Schally, A., Effect of somatostatin analogues on gastric and pancreatic secretion, Proc. Soc. Exptl. Biol. Med., 155,519, 1977.

365. Garsky, V., Clark, D., and Grant, N., Synthesis of a nonreducible cyclic analog of somatostatin having only growth hormone release inhibiting activity, Biochem. Biophys. Res. Commun., 73,911, 1976.

366. Ferland, L., Labrie, F., Coy, D., Arimura, A., and Schally, A., Inhibition by six somatostatin analogues of plasma growth hormone levels stimulated by thiamylal and morphine in the rat, Mol. Cell Endocrinol., 4,79, 1976.

367. Ohashi, S., Sawano, S., Kokubu, T., Gondo, M., and Sakakibara, K., Biologic activities of tyrosine-containing somatostatin analogs on inhibition of secretion of thyrotropin and growth hormone, Endocrinol. Jap., 23,435, 1976.

368. Holladay, L., and Puett, D., Somatostatin confirmation: Evidence for a stable intramolecular structure from circular dichroism, diffusion, and sedimentation equilibrium, Proc. Natl. Acad. Sci. USA, 73,1199, 1976.

369. Lien, E., Fenichel, R., Grant, N., Boxill, G., Greenwood, J., and Yardley, J., Prolonged suppression of pituitary and pancreatic hormone release by a somatostatin analog, Biochem. Biophys. Res. Commun., 77,1317, 1977.

370. Lien, E., Greenwood, J., and Sarantakis, D., Treatment of streptozotocin-diabetic dogs with a long-acting somatostatin analog, Diabetes, 288,491, 1979.

371. Bloom, S., Adrian, T., Barnes, A., Long, R., Hanley, J., Mallinson, C., Rivier, J., and Brown, M., New specific long-acting somatostatin analogues in the treatment of pancreatic endocrine tumors, Gastroenterology, 74,1013, 1978, (Abstract).

372. Arison, B., Hirschman, R., and Veber, D., Inferences about the confirmation of somatostatin at a biologic receptor based on NMR studies, Bioorganic Chem., 7,447, 1978.

373. Veber, D., Holly, F., Nult, R., Bergstrand, S., Brady, S., and Hirschman, R., Highly active cyclic and bicyclic somatostatin analogues of reduced ring size, Nature, 280,512, 1979.

3. BOTANICAL SOURCES OF FERTILITY REGULATING AGENTS: CHEMISTRY AND PHARMACOLOGY

A.S. Bingel & N.R. Farnsworth

I. **Introduction...150**

II. **Estrogenic Plants...151**
A. Isoflavonoids and coumestans 151; B. Miroestrol 155

III. **Fertility Control in the Female...156**
A. Antiovulatory agents 157; B. Interception 157; C. Abortifacients 169

IV. **Vaginal Contraceptives...179**

V. **Fertility Control in the Male...184**

VI. **Discussion...193**
A. Plant factors 195; B. Investigator factors 199; C. Observer factors 200, D. Conclusions 202

References...205

I. INTRODUCTION

Virtually every pharmacologic class of drug includes a natural product prototype, most frequently plant derived, which exhibits the classic effects of the pharmacologic category in question.[1] Thus, it would not be very surprising if the plant kingdom were also to prove a source of naturally occurring fertility regulating agents. Indeed, we cited over 1,300 plant species that might have such activity based on their folkloric reputation, on their chemical constituents, and/or on the results of their testing in animals.[2,3] Since then, we have gathered similar information concerning more than 2,000 additional species which might possibly have fertility regulating effects.[4] Space, of course, necessitates a limitation on the number of plants we can discuss.

This review presents a discussion of (a) the types of antifertility effect that have been demonstrated, tentatively or otherwise, to be produced by various plant species and (b) the problems[5] that unfortunately are associated with the evaluation and interpretation both of folkloric reports concerning fertility regulating plants and of studies reporting experimental results obtained with such plants. To illustrate the various components of these major points, we have selected for discussion throughout, specific genera, species, and/or phytochemical classes of compound, concerning which a reasonably substantial amount of literature has been published.

We should first point out, however, that the most popular, reversible means of contraception in use in the world today,[6] the oral hormonal contraceptives, are products, the majority of which contain estrogens and progestogens that are derived by partial synthesis from steroidal precursors obtained from plants,[7] specifically diosgenin from *Dioscorea* species (Dioscoreaceae) and stigmasterol from *Glycine max* (Leguminosae). Strictly speaking, these compounds merely represent starting materials, rather than botanicals which already possess significant fertility regulating activity. The reader, therefore, is referred to other sources,[6-11] and references therein, for information concerning steroidal contraceptives.

II. ESTROGENIC PLANTS

Plants which possess estrogenic activity, due predominantly to *non*-steroidal compounds, are nevertheless perhaps the first to come to mind when one is considering botanical sources of fertility regulating agents. Estrogens are able to prevent ovulation and were the sole antifertility component of the formerly available sequential oral contraceptives;[12] estrogens in high doses, furthermore, can prevent implantation in women (*vide infra*).[13] Of course, whether or not the presence of phytoestrogens could account for antifertility effects attributed ethnomedically, *i.e.* in folklore, to plants which have not yet been investigated in the laboratory remains unknown.

A. Isoflavonoids and coumestans

On the other hand, that infertility can occur in Australian ewes as a result of their grazing on clover [*e.g.* *Trifolium subterraneum* L. (Leguminosae)] pastures high in phytoestrogen content has been shown through numerous studies, many of which were reviewed recently by Livingston.[14] Although a number of alterations detrimental to reproduction may be induced by phytoestrogens, *e.g.* structural[15] and functional[16] changes in the hypothalamus, it appears that the failure of ewes to become pregnant in spite of repeated matings with fertile rams may be due most importantly to the failure of adequate numbers of sperm to enter the cervix following mating.[17] In ruminants, the cervix importantly serves as a reservoir from which sperm migrate to the uterus and thence to the oviducts, for a prolonged period following mating;[18] the properties of normal cervical mucus, *i.e.* the parallel alignment of its mucoid molecules which provides pathways for sperm to follow, enable this secretion to ensure the establishment of an adequate reservoir of sperm in the cervix. In ewes with clover disease, however, the amount of mucus secreted at estrus is greater than normal, and it is also thinner and more watery;[19] associated with the greater fluidity seems to be a decreased molecular anisotropy of the mucus, in turn preventing the normal orientation and progression of sperm within the cervix, as well as exposing them to phagocytic leukocytes. Adams[20] indeed found that sperm tended to swim in all directions in mucus obtained from clover affected ewes, this lack of orientation and of forward progression of sperm correlating with a statistically significant decrease in the spinnbarkeit of the mucus.

Of the various isoflavonoids and coumestans found in numerous plant species,[3] the ones studied most extensively in relation to clover disease are the isoflavones biochanin A (I), genistein (II), formononetin (IV), and daidzein (V), and the coumestan, coumestrol (VII) (see Figure 1). Besides occurring naturally in plants, II and V are produced as metabolites of I and IV, respectively, in the rumen of sheep. Most importantly with respect to clover induced infertility, V is metabolized further to equol (VI), an estrogenically active metabolite which is not further degraded.[21] In contrast, II is further metabolized to *p*-ethylphenol (III) which is estrogenically inactive; VII likewise appears to be inactivated in the sheep.

The determination of estrogenicity of these and other plant constituents typically has been based on their ability to cause an increase in uterine weight in ovariectomized or immature animals, even though such an effect is not entirely specific for estrogens.[22] On such a basis, VII has been found to be about 160 times less potent than the steroid, estradiol (VIII),[23] II even less potent, and I and IV less potent yet.[24] More recently, the activity

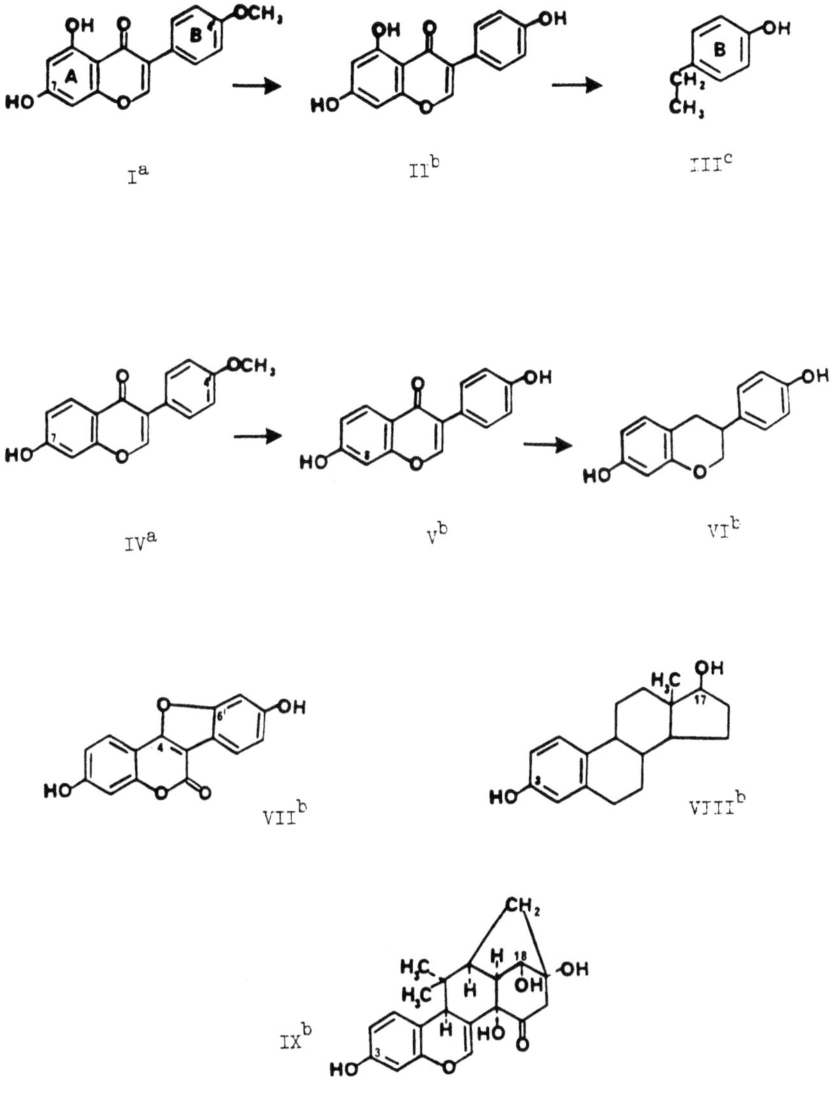

FIG. 1: Structural Comparison among Estrogenically Active and Estrogenically Inactive Compounds (I-IX).

See text for discussion and identification of compounds.

[a] Active *in vivo* after demethylation; inactive *in vitro*.

[b] Active *in vivo* and *in vitro*.

[c] Inactive *in vivo* and *in vitro*.

of such compounds has been examined *in vitro*; *i.e.* the ability of various plant estrogens to compete with estradiol-17β for binding sites on rabbit[23] and sheep[24] uterine cytosol receptors has been studied, and their relative binding affinities determined. Their low binding affinities correlated with their weak *in vivo* potencies. The data, furthermore, supported the idea that the *in vivo* "activity" of I and IV might actually be due to the activity of the 4'-demethylated metabolites, II, V, and VI; *i.e.* free 7- and 4'-hydroxyl groups, separated notably by a distance similar to that separating the 3- and 17-hydroxyl groups of VIII, apparently are necessary for significant binding to the estrogen receptor.[23]

If present *in vivo* at sufficiently high concentrations, weakly active phytoestrogens could be expected to exhibit a significant estrogenic effect,[21] and thus might inhibit fertility as did the previously available sequential oral contraceptives.[12] However, fertility impairment alternatively might result from an *antiestrogenic* effect of the phytoestrogen;[25] the latter might be present at a sufficient concentration to displace the more potent endogenous estrogens from their receptor sites in estrogen sensitive tissues,[21] yet be unable to substitute adequately for the displaced estrogen. Folman and Pope[25] demonstrated additive effects of weak and potent estrogens at low doses and antagonistic effects at high doses. Results of further studies[26] indicated that the interaction between weak and potent estrogens in estrogen sensitive tissues involved competition for retention at receptor sites followed by expression of the activity characteristic of the compound that was retained. That phytoestrogens could exert significant pharmacologic (be it estrogenic or antiestrogenic) activity *in vivo* is supported by the finding that such compounds have very low affinity for sex hormone binding globulin (SHBG)[27] and hence presumably circulate largely in a free, and therefore active, form; estradiol, in contrast, circulates largely in an inactive form due in part to its avid binding to SHBG.[28] One final point which may emphasize the importance of an *anti*estrogenic mechanism for the isoflavonoids and coumestans is the observation that fertility and sperm production in rams grazing estrogenic pastures do not seem to be impaired;[21] such impairment would be likely in males exposed to significant quantities of potent estrogens.[29]

B. Miroestrol

In contrast to the weakly active isoflavone and coumestan phytoestrogens, miroestrol (IX), isolated from the tuberous roots of *Pueraria mirifica* (Leguminosae), a woody, climbing plant found in northern Thailand,[30] has been found to be relatively similar in potency to VIII,[31,32] minor variations in relative potencies reported probably being related to differences among assay procedures and/or strains of test animals used. Jones and Pope,[31] furthermore, reported that IX could prevent implantation in rats, an effect characteristically shown by estrogens. Structure-activity-relationships among several of the compounds shown in Figure 1 have been discussed[23,24,32-35] in an attempt to explain their respective potencies. The somewhat greater potency of VII, relative to II, for example, has been attributed to the fact that the ring system of VII is held rigidly in one plane, thus approximating to the shape of VIII;[23] in contrast, since II lacks the 4,6' oxygen bridge, one of its phenolic rings is free to rotate. The structure of IX also is obviously quite rigid. In addition, the distance between the 3- and 18-hydroxyl groups of IX is reported to be 10.57 Å,[33] close to that expected between the 3- and 17-hydroxyl groups of VIII.

The estrogenic potency of IX reported experimentally supports the folkloric information concerning its source, *P. mirifica*. This plant was reported to "rejuvenate" old men and women,[34] which effect apparently included the induction of breast development and vaginal bleeding in women 60-80 years of age;[35] young people, furthermore, were not supposed to ingest this plant.[34]

Estrogenic effects of IX have also been demonstrated clinically, but only on a limited basis.[34] Vaginal cornification, withdrawal bleeding, breast enlargement and tenderness, nipple pigmentation, diminution of post-menopausal hot flushes, and side effects such as headache, nausea, and vomiting were among the phenomena inconsistently observed in a small number of amenorrheic women treated orally with one or five mg doses of IX daily for short periods of time.

A related species, *Pueraria tuberosa*, is distributed throughout much of India.[36] Its tubers are reported to be used for birth control by nomads in the J and K State and as supplementary food by certain tribes of Assam, among whom population density appears to be low. Although the isolation of IX from *P. tuberosa* has not been reported, its roots do contain the weak estrogen, V, and two 8-*C*-glycosides of the latter, puerarin and puerarin 4',6"-diacetate.[37] Data from some preliminary and only partially controlled experiments suggest that *P. tuberosa* may have estrogenic and antifertility effects;[36] extracts of the plant appeared to promote an increase in uterine weight in immature rats and to interfere with early pregnancy in adult rats. Finally, although a variety of pharmacologic agents besides estrogens can cause galactorrhea by inhibiting prolactin inhibitory factor (PIF),[38] it is interesting to note that *P. tuberosa* has also been reported to be used as a galactagogue.[36]

III. FERTILITY CONTROL IN THE FEMALE

Plants to be discussed in this section are ones investigated for systemic use in females for the purpose of (a) preventing conception, *i.e.* preventing, by direct or indirect mechanisms, the successful implantation of a blastocyst in the uterine lining,[39] or (b) inducing abortion. As will be seen (B. Interception), dosage regimens sometimes are such that this distinction may become less clear.

A. Antiovulatory agents

From among the large number of plants reportedly associated with fertility regulation,[4] relatively few have been investigated for antiovulatory activity, perhaps because of the availability of the highly efficacious combination type oral contraceptives which act importantly, although not exclusively, by inhibiting the hypothalamus, and consequently ovulation.[10] The combination type oral contraceptives induce a pharmacologic, not physiologic, state,[11] but nevertheless their dosage regimen is such that an artificial withdrawal bleeding regularly occurs.

Amenorrhea, in contrast, is the more likely, and not necessarily desirable result when hypothalamic inhibition is achieved by agents which lack estrogenic and progestogenic activity;[12] amenorrhea associated with anovulation has been reported, for example, in rhesus monkeys treated with reserpine and in women treated with synthetic phenothiazines. In Table 1 are listed a few examples of natural products which have been shown to interfere with hypothalamic-hypophyseal-ovarian function. Although their other more predominant pharmacologic effects prevent their use as ovulation inhibitors, the presence of such compounds in these or related plants could account for antifertility effects that might be attributed to them.

The method typically employed in screening plants for antiovulatory activity is that in which extracts are tested for the ability to prevent the occurrence of copper induced ovulation in the rabbit.[42]

B. Interception

An ideal method of fertility control might involve (a) the use of an

Table 1. Natural Products Capable of Interfering with Hypothalamic-Hypophyseal-Ovarian Function.

Product	Source	Species	Reference
Reserpine	*Rauvolfia serpentina* Benth. (Apocynaceae)	Rhesus monkey, human	12
Morphine	*Papaver somniferum* (Papaveraceae)	Rat, human	40 and references therein
Atropine [(±)-hyoscyamine]	*Atropa belladonna* *Datura stramonium* (Solanaceae)	Rat	41

agent postcoitally to ensure the prevention of implantation if fertilization were to occur and/or (b) the use of an agent just prior to one's expected menses to ensure the occurrence of menstruation even if implantation had occurred.[43] High dose estrogens and intravaginally administered prostaglandins notwithstanding, such ideals have not been met; consequently, many of the investigations of plants which might have fertility regulating effects are directed primarily toward identifying those which may prevent implantation and/or interfere with the continuance of early pregnancy. Unfortunately, some confusion of terminology exists in the literature, such confusion being accentuated further by the various dosage regimens used.

Morris and van Wagenen,[44] and subsequently others,[45,46] used the term "interception" specifically to refer to the use of high doses of estrogens to *prevent* the occurrence of implantation in women exposed to unprotected coitus close to the time of ovulation. Naqvi and Warren,[47] however, employed the term "interceptive" to avoid using the term "abortifacient," which to them, in 1971, connoted surgical intervention. Their experiments, in fact, specifically involved the administration of potentially abortifacient drugs to rats beginning on Day 7 of pregnancy, a full day *after* implantation had been completed.

Likewise, Pakrashi and coworkers[48-52] have used "interception" to describe the antifertility effects they reported for extracts and/or constituents of *Aristolochia indica* L. (Aristolochiaceae) administered to mice *after* the day of implantation, and in definite contradistinction to the "antiimplantation" effects they reported when the mice were dosed *prior* to implantation.[50] Although these workers have used the words "interceptive" and "abortifacient" interchangeably,[49,50,53] they have also reported on the interceptive *and* abortifacient activity of *A. indica*,[54] apparently distinguishing in the latter study between dosing at or just after the time of implantation *versus* dosing at or after midpregnancy.

A cursory look at their entire series of papers,[48-57] which also present a few data obtained on rats,[54] hamsters,[54] and rabbits,[56] would lead one to believe that several of the numerous constituents isolated from the roots of *A. indica*[58] might indeed possess antifertility activity, although one's curiosity is aroused by data reporting that antifertility effects were seen in 55.5%,[50] 63.6%,[50] and 75%,[55] respectively, of groups containing *10* mice each. Nevertheless, since *A. indica* has a folkloric reputation for possessing fertility regulating properties,[2] and contains a cytotoxic constituent, aristolochic acid,[3] a further, adequately controlled look at the pre- and/or postimplantational activity of *p*-coumaric acid (X),[51,52] aristolic acid (XI),[56,57] aristolic acid methyl ester (XII),[53] and the uncharacterized sesquiterpene (m.p. 150°C)[50,55] might be worthwhile.

Chandhoke,[59] and coworkers,[60] in contrast, used a Days 1-7 dosage regimen, thus dosing their rats during both pre- and postimplantational periods; in their discussions of the antifertility effects they reported for daturalactone (DQ_1) (XIII) [*Datura quercifolia* HBK. (Solanaceae)][59] and for the waxy alkaloid of *Piper* species (Piperaceae),[60] "interceptive" was referred to synonymously with "antiimplantation" and with "antiimplantation/early abortifacient," respectively. More precisely defined activities may actually not be possible; Chandhoke's data[59] indicated that dosing for the full seven days seemed to be necessary for maximum inhibition of pregnancy.

Complicating the interpretation of such studies even further, particularly with respect to their potential extrapolation to the human, is the observation that the effects seen may sometimes be attributed to estrogenicity; DQ_1, for example, seems to be weakly estrogenic.[61] Estrogens appear

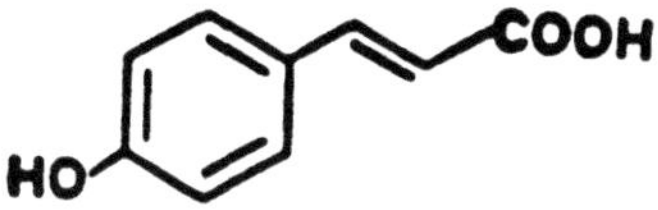

X

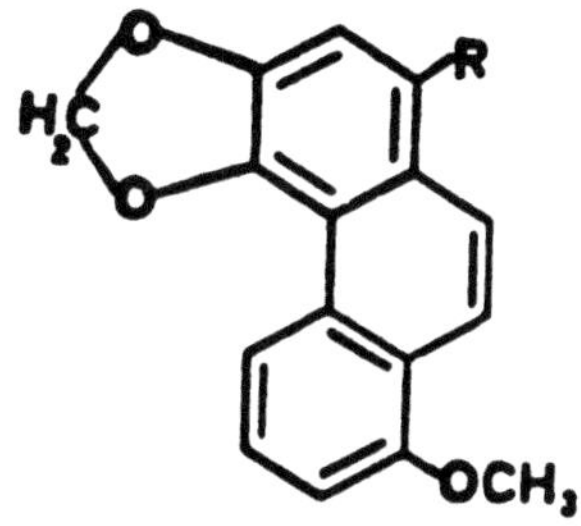

XI R=COOH
XII R=COOCH$_3$

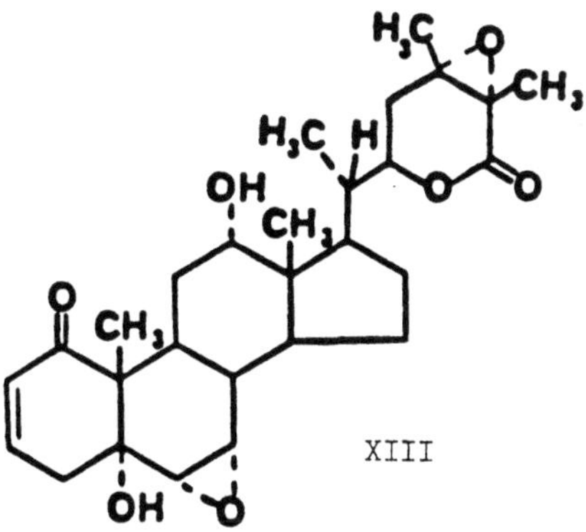

XIII

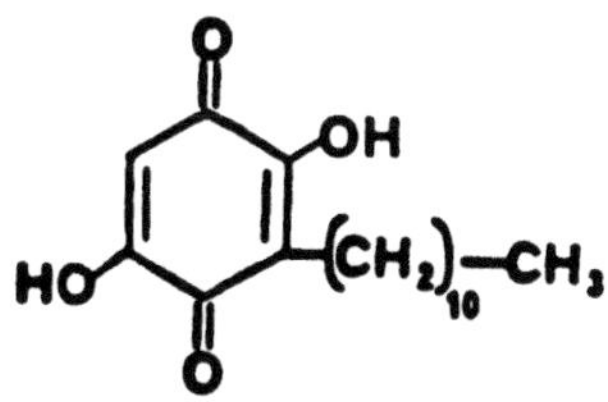

XIV

FIG. 2: Plant constituents (X-XIV) reputed to have antifertility effects when administered postcoitally.

to be universally active in *preventing* implantation[62] and apparently also can interrupt pregnancy in rabbits,[63] rats,[64] and hamsters,[64] but not in humans[63] or rhesus monkeys,[63] when administered *after* implantation has occurred. The possibility that antiestrogenic effects may be demonstrated by weak estrogens[21,25,62] must also be kept in mind when one is confronted with reports that plant extracts seemingly active postcoitally also appear to be antiestrogenic.

Kholkute and Udupa demonstrated antiestrogenic activity in the total alcohol and total benzene extracts of *Hibiscus rosa-sinensis* L. (Malvaceae) flowers,[65] and subsequently showed that the latter extract could also exert antifertility effects when administered postcoitally.[66] The pregnancy inhibition in this case seems to have been the result of the extract's antiestrogenic action since pregnancy was *not* inhibited when estrogen was administered in addition.[66] Specifically, the total benzene extract of *H. rosa-sinensis* flowers effectively interrupted pregnancy in rats when administered orally from Days 1-10 at a dose of 250 mg/kg. Although some effect was seen when the rats were treated only on Days 1-6 or 4-6, no significant effect occurred when treatment was carried out only on Days 1-3. In rats being treated on Days 1-10, the simultaneous administration of estrone (1 mcg/day s.c.) was able to counteract the antifertility effect of the extract, presumably by supplying exogenously the estrogen needed for implantation. Whereas estrogen seems to be necessary for implantation in rats and mice,[2] it apparently is not necessary for implantation in rabbits, guinea pigs, and hamsters, and is considered to be of doubtful necessity in humans;[62] therefore, the relevance of Kholkute and Udupa's observations[66] to the fertility regulating folkloric reputation of *H. rosa-sinensis* is unclear.

The results of additional studies by these[67,68] and other[69] workers lend further support to the idea that the benzene extract of the flowers of this plant indeed exerts postcoital antifertility effects in rats. Attempts to isolate the active constituent(s), however, have been unsuccessful.[70] Quercetin, cyanidin, and hentriacontane, isolated from the total benzene extract, were each inactive in inhibiting pregnancy in rats even when given at a dose 10 times that at which the crude extract was administered.

The flowers of *Butea monosperma* (Leguminosae), also known as *Butea frondosa*,[71] may possess fertility regulating activity not explainable by estrogenicity or antiestrogenicity; Tewari and coworkers,[72] for example, presented data indicating that powdered *B. monosperma* flowers were not estrogenic in rats at a dose of 2 gm/kg. Doses of 200 mg/kg of an alcohol extract of the petals of *B. monosperma* given orally on Days 1-5 exerted antifertility effects in rats.[73] Although other data[74] suggested that this alcohol concentrate might be weakly antiestrogenic, a crystalline fraction of the extract, reported to have no estrogenic or antiestrogenic activity, was similarly effective postcoitally at a dose of only 30 mg/kg;[73] unfortunately, the actual uterine weight data supporting the lack of estrogenic/antiestrogenic effects for the crystalline fraction were not presented.

Embelia ribes Burm. f. (Myrsinaceae) and its constituent, embelin (XIV), have been tested for postcoital antifertility activity in rats under various dosage regimens, as summarized in Table 2. It should be noted that no rats were dosed with the seed extract on Days 14-16, only. Therefore, the possibility cannot be ruled out that the resorptions found on Day 18 might actually have resulted from an effect of the second series of doses added onto an effect of the first series, the earlier effect not having been discernible on Day 10. This possibility is supported by the report[78] of an increased incidence of stillborn pups within relatively normal sized litters, when rats were

Table 2. Effects of *Embelia ribes* and Embelin Administered Orally to Rats

Preparation	Dosage Regimen[a]	Pregnancy Inhibition[b]	Reference
Powdered roots	100 mg/kg Days 1-7	+	75
Seeds			76
50% ethanol extract	200 mg/kg Days 1-7 PLUS 200 mg/kg Days 14-16	- +[c]	
Powdered berries			77
Water extract	100 mg/kg Days 1-5	+	
Alcohol extract	100 mg/kg Days 1-5	+	
Petroleum ether extract	100 mg/kg Days 1-5	-	
Powdered berries			78
Methanol extract	60 or 120 mg Days 1-7	-	
Petroleum ether extract	25 or 50 mg Days 1-7	-	
Embelin	0.3, 3, or 30 mg Days 1-7	-	78
Embelin	10 mg/kg Days 1-5	+	79
Embelin	15 or 30 mg/kg Days 1-5	±	80
Embelin	60 or 120 mg/kg Days 1-5	+	80

[a] Day 1 = Day on which sperm were found in the vaginal smear.

[b] Data were based on between six and 12 rats per dosage regimen; no corresponding control data were presented in the first two references cited in this table.

[c] Resorption (Day 18) of implantation sites that had been present on Day 10.

treated on Days 1-7 with the higher dose of both the methanol and petroleum ether extracts of powdered berries. Arora and coworkers[77] also reported having tested Maswin tablets, reputed to have been prepared from the aqueous extract of *E. ribes* berries. Interestingly, this preparation prevented implantation in 16/20 rats at a dose of 400 mg/kg given orally on Days 1-5, but was inactive at doses of 80 and 200 mg/kg.

Rathinam and coworkers[79] could not demonstrate any estrogenic or antiestrogenic activity for embelin at a dose of 10 mg/kg whereas Radhakrishnan and Alam[81] concluded that embelin was antiestrogenic at a dose of 120 mg/kg; the number of animals used in the latter study, and the variation in response among them, were not indicated, however.

A possible estrogenic effect of 50% ethanol and benzene extracts of *E. ribes* berries, additive to that of estrone (0.1 mcg), seems to have been demonstrated by Prakash[82] when either extract was administered orally to ovariectomized, immature rats that were also receiving the steroid; no animals were treated with either extract alone, however. In contrast, 100 mg/kg p.o. doses of an aqueous extract of *E. ribes* berries were reported to be antiestrogenic in intact, immature rats simultaneously injected with 0.1 mcg estradiol s.c.[77] A possible hormonal or antihormonal effect, whether direct or indirect, of *E. ribes* is further suggested by observations in intact adult rats. Oral administration of 50% ethanol and benzene extracts of *E. ribes* berries appeared to interfere with estrous cyclicity,[83] and the feeding of the powdered berries, as well as the oral administration of extracts of these berries, interfered with mating behavior;[78] both cyclicity and mating in rats, of course, are importantly dependent on normal hormonal interrelationships.[2] It is interesting to note, however, that Kholkute *et al.*,[78] after extensively discussing the "antifertility" effects (≥ 50% "inhibition of pregnancy") they had observed after treating their rats prior to and during their pairing with males, finally mention, almost as an afterthought, that the antifertility effects were apparently due to a lack of mating! Except as a possible demonstration of interference with the normal hormonal milieu, the relevance to humans of observations that plants exert antifertility effects by preventing mating, is unclear. Curiously, when Kholkute and coworkers[84] later cited this study, they made reference only to the "antifertility," not antimating, effects they had observed in their *E. ribes* treated rats.

Other plants have been reported to interfere with mating in mice,[85] as well as in rats;[86,87] this effect must therefore be considered when one sees reports of antifertility activity of plants administered to animals *during* the period of pairing, if no mention is made of either vaginal plugs or sperm in vaginal smears having been observed.

The plant species so far discussed in this section represent only a very small proportion of the numerous species which have been tested, largely in India, for postcoital activity in rodents; preliminary data concerning a number of these have recently been summarized.[75,76] Despite the folkloric fertility regulating reputation of these plants, few have been demonstrated to have such activity in the laboratory. Although species differences, rat *versus* human, could be one explanation, as could the fact that only relatively rarely are reputed fertility regulating plants specifically cited as being used *after intercourse*,[4] a closer look at papers cited by Garg *et al.*,[75] for example, reveals that testing often seems to have been inadequate either to support or negate the possibility that the plants examined might have fertility regulating activity. Various extracts, and fractions thereof, frequently have been administered, at one or more dosage levels, to as few as five rats per group,[88-99] with the results often ranging between two and four rats pregnant per group of five; data for vehicle treated control groups, furthermore, often are lacking.[88-95]

Workers[59,60,66,77,80] have reported less than 100% fertility in control groups; furthermore, there are reports[100-104] of plants being used to *promote* fertility. Khanna and coworkers[89] have argued that the "negative" results they had obtained with some of their plants were an indication that their suspending agent did not possess antifertility activity; presumably that justified to them that the use of vehicle treated controls was unnecessary. However, since vehicle control data were not obtained, the possibility cannot be ruled out that their plants might have possessed fertility *promoting* effects. Consequently, the nonuse of vehicle treated controls in studies involving potential fertility regulating agents remains unjustified.

More recently, Garg[105-107] has reported on the postcoital effects of a number of plant extracts, virtually all of which were tested in groups consisting of 10 rats each. Although the number of control animals (10) was still quite small relative to the total number of extract treated rats in each study (162, 270, and 60, respectively), the data were such that further investigation of postcoital antifertility effects of the following should be considered warranted: the petroleum ether, alcohol, and aqueous extracts of *Daucus carota* L. (Umbelliferae) seeds and of *Curcuma longa* L. (Zingiberaceae) rhizomes; the alcohol and aqueous extracts of *Cuminum cyminum* L. (Umbelliferae) seeds; and the alcohol extract of *Hyptis suaveolens* Poit. (Labiatae) leaves.

Dosage regimens in which rats are treated both before and after the normal time of implantation, appear to be most commonly employed in studies aimed at identifying plants which may exert postcoital antifertility effects.[4] As already discussed, plants possessing sufficient estrogenicity should show activity in the laboratory under such regimens. However, plants possessing cytotoxic properties may also demonstrate effectiveness under such regimens.[108] Some antimetabolites, for example, seem to be particularly effective in interrupting pregnancy in rats when administered shortly after implantation,[109] although some degree of effectiveness could be demonstrated for several compounds given either prior to implantation, or at midpregnancy.

The antimitotic agent, desacetylmethylcolchicine [*Colchicum* sp. (Liliaceae)], was completely effective in interrupting pregnancy in rabbits at doses of 0.5-5 mg/kg s.c. injected on Day 12, but relatively ineffective at such doses administered on Days 2 or 5.[110] Another antimitotic agent, podophyllotoxin [*Podophyllum peltatum* (Berberidaceae)], at a dose of 0.25 mg, was reported to interrupt pregnancy in mice when injected subcutaneously on Days 3, 6, 12, or 14,[111] but was relatively ineffective when administered on Day 1. These antimitotics also disrupted pregnancy in rats when injected intraperitoneally at various times after implantation;[112,113] effects of earlier dosing were not determined. Toxicity appears to have been exerted directly on the fetuses,[110,112,113] and apparently no significant effects on the placentae could be demonstrated.

A third antimitotic agent, vinblastine [*Catharanthus roseus* (Apocynaceae)], effectively disrupted pregnancy in rabbits at doses of 0.3 mg/kg i.v. injected on Days 1, 7, 14, and 28;[110] single doses of 0.5 mg/kg i.v. injected before implantation were somewhat less effective. Vinblastine also disrupted pregnancy in rats at doses of 0.12-0.30 mg/kg i.p. injected on Days 7-12.[114]

The usefulness of such cytotoxic agents for interrupting pregnancy is limited, however, both by their potential toxicity to the maternal organism as well as by their potential for producing teratogenic effects in the surviving fetuses when given in marginal doses or at marginal times.[108] Vinblastine, vincristine (*C. roseus*), and colchicine (*Colchicum* sp.), administered after implantation, have produced teratogenic, as well as fetocidal, effects in the hamster,[115] as have vincristine, colchicine, and maytansine [*Maytenus* sp. (Celastraceae)] in the mouse,[116] desacetylmethylcolchicine in the rabbit,[110] and vinblastine in the rat.[114] The relative lack of efficacy, and the possibility of teratogenicity in the case of failure, thus preclude the use of known cytotoxic agents for terminating pregnancy in the human.[108] On the other hand, the presence of cytotoxic constituents could account for the antifertility effects attributed folklorically to some plants;[3] Schvartzman *et al.*[117] have discussed, for example, the possibility that the antimitotic activity of *Aristolochia triangularis* Cham. might contribute to its reputed abortifacient effect.

C. Abortifacients

In 1975,[2] we cited over 600 species of plant for which there were folkloric information and/or experimental data suggesting their potential usefulness as abortifacients. Subsequently,[5] we discussed many of the difficulties involved both in interpreting the ethnomedical reports, and in correlating the experimental data, largely from *in vitro* studies, with their possible applicability to the *in vivo* situation.

Oxytocic drugs are used clinically to induce labor at term (*e.g.* oxytocin) and to control postpartum hemorrhage (*e.g.* ergonovine and methylergonovine),[118] but are not readily useful as abortifacients. The uterus is rather insensitive to oxytocin earlier in gestation,[119] even at relatively large doses.[118] Use of ergot alkaloids for labor induction, and presumably also for abortion induction, currently is precluded because in high doses they tend to increase resting tonus and to produce prolonged contractions.[118] Historically, however, abortion was reported to be a frequent complication of ergot (*Claviceps purpurea*) poisoning,[118] and ergot was employed for many years as a means of facilitating labor, though apparently with a resultant increase in the number of stillbirths. Thus, plants reported to expel the placenta, relieve postpartum bleeding, and/or promote difficult delivery[5] might possibly be able to induce abortion. To presume, however, that plants reported to promote menstruation or to be used for amenorrhea will be abortifacient implies that the lack of menstruation is due to pregnancy, which may or may not be true.[120] *Solanum bahamense* L. (Solanaceae) berries crushed in water, are reported to be drunk by women who have missed a menstrual period;[121] apparently, if the period has merely been delayed, the women will menstruate, but menstruation will not resume if they are pregnant.

Many plants have merely been reported to be abortifacient,[2,5] with no further details. Devereux[122] reported on the abortion practices of more than 300 primitive cultures, describing the method(s) employed by more than 200 of them. Although the majority of these tribes apparently used preparations of natural products, half of the latter tribes employed other methods in addition, which most frequently included mechanical means aimed at damaging the fetus through the abdominal wall. The use, or lack thereof, of other abortifacient methods is rarely, if ever, discussed in literature reporting plants reputed to have abortifacient properties; furthermore, the incidence of spontaneous abortion is estimated to be at least 25%,[123] when spontaneous termination of even the earliest gestations is also considered. Therefore, it becomes difficult to place much confidence in reports of abortifacient plants unless such reports are supported by experimental and/or clinical data, or unless perhaps the same plant species has been reported to be used for abortion in two or more geographically distant cultures or countries,[5] or at least by widely separated tribes.[124]

Many of the experimental data concerning potentially abortifacient plants represent the results of studies in which the ability of plant extracts (or isolated constituents thereof) to stimulate uterine muscle contractions, has been examined *in vitro*. Although the hormone, oxytocin, can serve as an excellent standard[125] against which plant extracts may be screened for *in vitro* uterine stimulant activity, its lack of efficacy as an *in vivo* abortifacient must be kept in mind as one peruses the long list of plants for which *in vitro* uterine stimulant activity has been reported.[2]

An absolute ethanol extract of the dry, powdered rhizomes of *Gloriosa superba* L. (Liliaceae), for example, reportedly stimulated the following uterine preparations *in vitro*: pregnant and nonpregnant guinea pig, pregnant and nonpregnant rabbit, nonpregnant dog, and nonpregnant human;[126] pregnant and nonpregnant rat uteri, however, were not responsive. More importantly, abortion could not be induced by this extract given orally to rabbits in doses of 1.13, 113, or 11,300 mcg/kg at eight hour intervals on Days 10 and 11 of pregnancy.

A second example of lack of correlation between *in vitro* and *in vivo* results involves plumbagin (XV) and its source, *Plumbago zeylanica* L. (Plumbaginaceae) roots.[127] Ko[128] examined the *in vitro* effects of plumbagin on pregnant and nonpregnant rabbit and guinea pig uteri; low doses typically produced stimulation and high doses, paralysis. Bhatia and Lal[127] obtained similar results with the same types of isolated preparation treated with plumbagin itself or with either a decoction or tincture of *P. zeylanica* roots. The latter workers, however, could not induce abortion in pregnant rabbits or guinea pigs either with small or with large, mildly toxic doses of plumbagin, or of *P. zeylanica* decoction, administered orally, intravenously, or subcutaneously. Premakumari and coworkers,[129] in contrast, reported plumbagin to be abortifacient in rats. Their criterion, however, and the only evidence reported, was the appearance of vaginal bleeding between Days 8-14 of pregnancy; exactly how this bleeding was distinguished from the bloody placental sign often apparent in the vaginal smear of rodents at mid- to late pregnancy,[130] was not explained.

Leonurus artemisia (Lour.) S.Y. Hu (Labiatae) has long been used as a remedy in Chinese folk medicine.[131] Included among its reported effects are alleviation of menstrual pains, correction of amenorrhea, facilitation of difficult labor, expulsion of dead fetus or placenta, and stoppage of postpartum hemorrhage.[132] It has also been suggested, although without direct evidence, that *L. artemisia*[132] and/or leonurine (XVI),[133] (a uterotonic principle isolated from this plant[134,135] and recently synthesized[136]) might prove useful in inducing abortion. The actual data reported merely indicate a stimulant action for a crude extract of *L. artemisia* on nonpregnant rabbit,[132,133] rat,[132,133] and human[132,135] uteri *in vitro*, and for leonurine itself on nonpregnant rat uterus *in vitro*[134,135] and *in situ*.[136]

Folkloric use of aqueous decoctions of *Oldenlandia affinis* DC. (Rubiaceae), as regards the reproductive system, seems to be restricted to the acceleration of childbirth among tribes in the Kasai province of Zaïre and in the Central African Republic.[137] Gran isolated a polypeptide (m.w. *ca.* 4,000) from the aboveground parts of this plant,[138] and reported that this peptide could produce contractions in isolated preparations of estrogenized rat, estrogenized rabbit, and pregnant human uteri *in vitro*;[124] uterine contractions similarly were produced *in situ* when the peptide was administered by catheter directly into the peritoneal cavity of rats. In contrast, action of this peptide on estrogenized rabbit and proestrous rat uteri *in situ*, following intravenous administration, was weak and inconsistent, although

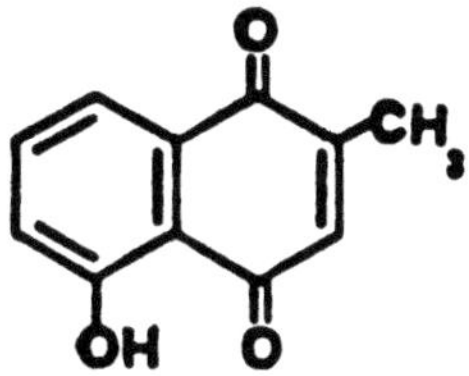

XV

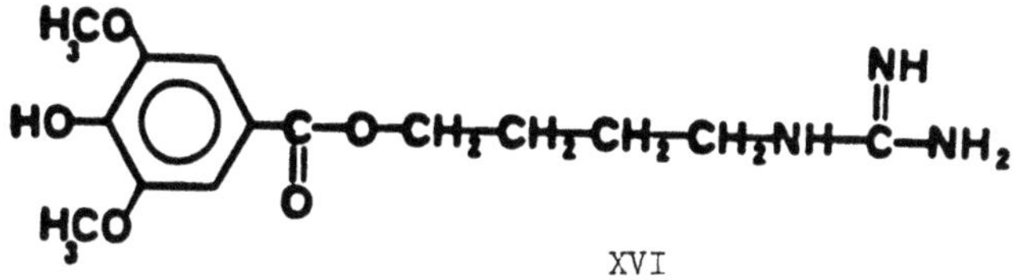

XVI

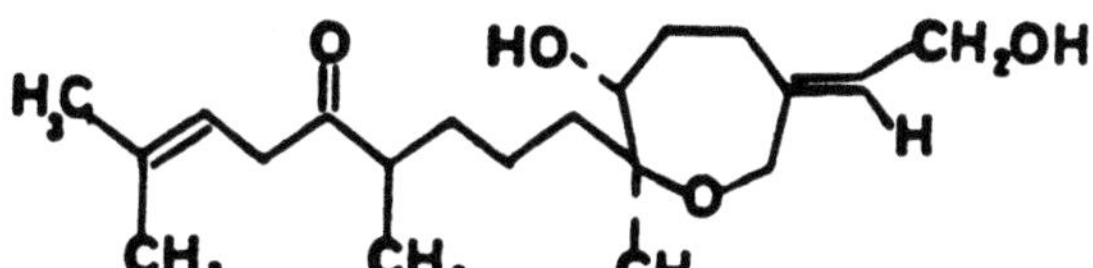

XVII

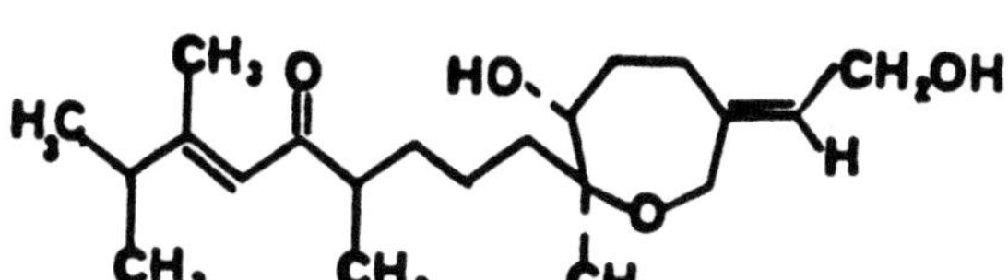

XVIII

FIG. 3: Plant constituents (XV-XVIII) reported to possess uterine stimulant activity.

deleterious effects were produced on the circulatory system. Intragastric administration of this peptide to rats and rabbits by stomach tube, however, produced no effect on either the uterus or on the circulatory system. This lack of any effect when the peptide was given enterally makes one question whether it could be responsible for the strong uterine contractions, short delivery time, and unfortunate cervical spasms reported to occur in African women drinking aqueous extracts of *O. affinis* during labor.[138] Although Gran pointed out that oxytocin (m.w. 1,007) can be administered buccally,[138] it remains to be demonstrated whether or not the considerably larger *O. affinis* peptide might possibly be absorbed through the buccal mucosa during *oral* dosing.

Interestingly, Gran[137,138] also isolated serotonin (5-hydroxytryptamine) from the aboveground parts of *O. affinis* and demonstrated the ability of this compound to produce contractions in isolated preparations of estrogenized rat uteri *in vitro*. Nevertheless, the contribution, if any, of the serotonin content to the childbirth accelerating activity reputedly possessed by *O. affinis* is unclear; Gran[124] reportedly found no uterine (or circulatory) reaction in rats or rabbits following the intragastric administration of either an aqueous extract of the plant, or serotonin itself. He pointed out, furthermore, that serotonin has been considered to be inactive if given orally[137] because of its being rapidly destroyed in the gastrointestinal tract.[138]

Extracts of *Albizia* species (Leguminosae) have been reported to be used by East African women to accelerate labor and to induce abortion.[139] The use of such native medicines during labor has been implicated, moreover, as a cause of uterine rupture in Ugandan women,[140] although the combination of their small, shallow pelvis and relatively large infants must be considered contributory as well. In 1959, Lipton[141] briefly summarized experimental results obtained with cold aqueous extracts of the dried bark of *Albizia gummifera* (Gmel.) C.A. Smith, *A. grandibracteata* Taub., and *A. chinensis* (Osbeck) Merr., reporting that these extracts produced contractions in pregnant mouse, rat, guinea pig, sheep, cow, and human uterine preparations *in vitro*, and in pregnant and nonpregnant monkey uteri *in situ* following intravenous administration; these extracts also reportedly induced partial or complete abortion in rats, rabbits, and guinea pigs.

From a methanol extract of the bark of *A. gummifera*, Lipton[139] subsequently isolated the active principle (apparently a mixture of saponins) which he named albitocin; hydrolysis products of albitocin included an unsaturated triterpene acid and four sugars: glucose, rhamnose, xylose, and arabinose. Available evidence[139,142,143] indicates that albitocin is responsible for the uterine effects reported experimentally for crude extracts of this plant.[141] Uterine contractions were produced by albitocin *in vitro*[139] and *in situ*;[142] variations in response, however, were found both among the various animal species employed and among their respective reproductive status.[139] Intragastric administration of up to 5 mg/kg albitocin, moreover, failed to produce uterine contractions *in situ* in pregnant guinea pigs,[142] although contractions did occur when a dose of 0.25 mg/kg was applied directly onto the exposed uterus. Intravenous administration of up to 8 mg/kg albitocin was reported to be effective in producing uterine contractions in pregnant and nonpregnant animals of several species, including the pregnant guinea pig.[142]

A large discrepancy was found between the ED50 enteral and parenteral abortifacient doses for albitocin in guinea pigs;[143] by gastric intubation, the ED50 was determined to be 11.0 mg/kg compared with 0.7 by the intraperitoneal route. The ED50 abortifacient doses by the intraperitoneal and/or intravenous route were also found to be low in mice, rats, rabbits, and monkeys, ranging between 0.5 and 3.2 mg/kg. The corresponding LD50 doses, unfortunately, were usually only barely higher than those required to induce abortion;[143] furthermore, albitocin appears to have caused renal tubular necrosis in rabbits and hepatic necrosis in rats and mice, toxicity apparently being less severe following oral dosing than after parenteral administration.

Tea prepared from the leaves of *Montanoa tomentosa* (Compositae) reportedly has been used in Mexico for centuries to induce menses and labor and to terminate early pregnancy.[144] This bitter tasting tea, brewed by boiling the leaves in water, apparently has been used not only by women who have merely missed a menstrual period, and therefore might be pregnant, but also by those who are frankly pregnant, for the purpose of terminating that condition.[145] The oral administration of semipurified leaf extracts of *M. tomentosa* to two women, 31 and 39 weeks pregnant, respectively, was followed by expulsion of the uterine contents approximately four hours later.[146] Oral administration of another such extract to a woman with an 11 week hydatidiform molar pregnancy was followed approximately 19 minutes later by the onset of uterine contractions; the latter lasted 12 hours, at the end of which time the uterine contents were expelled.

Two oxepane diterpenoids, zoapatanol (XVII) and montanol (XVIII), were recently isolated as oils, from an aqueous extract of the leaves of *M. tomentosa*.[144] Zoapatanol and montanol, at doses of 1-4 mg/kg i.v. and 25-40 mg/kg i.v., respectively, have been reported to produce contractions in rabbit uteri *in situ*;[145] zoapatanol, furthermore, was reported to interrupt pregnancy in guinea pigs, apparently by causing abortion or resorption, when administered at doses of 25-85 mg/kg i.p. on Day 22 of pregnancy. Further details are awaiting publication.[144]

As early as 1596, an extract of the root tuber of *Trichosanthes kirilowii*

Maxim. (Cucurbitaceae) was reported to be used in Chinese medicine for inducing menstruation and expelling fetal membranes,[147] although, curiously, it traditionally was applied externally. In 1976,[148] a report appeared concerning 200 cases in which midtrimester abortion or expulsion of a dead fetus was attempted by means of intramuscular administration of a crude extract of this tuber, at doses of 5-10 mg. The shortest injection to abortion interval was one and a half days, the longest, thirteen and a half; for 102 of the 198 successful inductions, the interval ranged between four and seven days. From the crude extract, prepared from juice squeezed from the fresh tuber,[147] the active component, trichosanthin, subsequently was isolated and characterized as a basic protein (m.w. *ca.* 18,000).[149] Additional studies involving mice,[150-152] rabbits,[153] and monkeys,[154,155] as well as humans,[156-160] have been carried out in an attempt to elucidate the site(s) and mechanism(s) of the abortifacient action of trichosanthin.

A ^{131}I labeled crude extract of the tuber, for example, administered to a small number of women undergoing midtrimester abortion, was shown to be absorbed slowly from an intramuscular injection site.[156] Radioactivity determinations following intraamniotic administration indicated that when given by this route, the extract tended to remain localized within the uterus; side effects reportedly were milder as well. Based on results with an indirect immunofluorescence technique in the mouse, it was concluded that trichosanthin acts directly on the placenta.[150] Day 10 pregnant mice were injected with trichosanthin at a dose of 2 mg i.v. or 0.2 mg s.c. and autopsied during the following 24 hour period. Fluorescence was observed in placental tissue but not in fetal tissue, except in nuclei of fetal erythrocytes in animals exposed to the high intravenous dose. The presence of necrotic degeneration in the same placental tissues was also reported. Placental specimens from rhesus monkeys which had been given trichosanthin, 1.4-4 mg i.m. or i.v. during mid- or late pregnancy, were examined by both light microscopy[154] and electron microscopy;[155] damage typically was seen in the syncytiotrophoblast, which structure is responsible for the secretion of chorionic gonadotropin, placental lactogen (chorionic somatomammotropin), estriol, and progesterone.[147] Serum levels of chorionic gonadotropin[157,160] and placental lactogen,[160] and urinary levels of pregnanediol[159] and estriol[159] were indeed shown to decrease following intramuscular or intraamniotic administration of trichosanthin preparations to women, for the induction of midtrimester abortion. Placental samples from other women undergoing surgical abortion were cultured *in vitro*;[158] exposure of these tissues to trichosanthin resulted in degeneration of the syncytiotrophoblast and inhibition of chorionic gonadotropin secretion.

Trichosanthin has been demonstrated to stimulate contractions of pregnant rabbit uteri *in situ* and to enhance the response of such uteri to oxytocin.[153] Administration of a synthetic progestogen, megestrol acetate, or of a prostaglandin biosynthesis inhibitor, indomethacin, tended to decrease the uterine response to trichosanthin. This evidence thus supports the hypotheses (a) that trichosanthin, by virtue of its deleterious effects on the syncytiotrophoblast, and the resultant decreased secretion of progesterone, may permit the uterus to become more sensitive to endogenous oxytocin, and (b) that trichosanthin may cause the production of endogenous prostaglandins which in turn stimulate uterine contractions, thus promoting abortion.[153] The abortifacient activity of trichosanthin administered to mice on Day 17 of pregnancy was decreased when aspirin, another prostaglandin synthesis inhibitor, was given repeatedly on Days 15-18;[151] administration of aspirin on Day 17 only, simultaneously with trichosanthin, did not interfere with the latter's activity, however.

The possibility that the allergenic properties of the crude extract of *T. kirilowii* tuber might contribute to the pregnancy terminating activity of the latter in mice seems to have been ruled out;[152] administration of an antihistamine, promethazine, to prevent hypersensitivity reactions to the trichosanthin preparation did not prevent fetal death. Fetal death apparently is the response seen in mice following midtrimester trichosanthin administration, rather than actual fetal expulsion as occurs in the human.[150]

IV. VAGINAL CONTRACEPTIVES

One of the oldest contraceptive techniques is that involving the precoital intravaginal application of various types of substance which might act as physical and/or chemical barriers to the passage of sperm.[161] Of the pharmacologically active vaginal contraceptives which are currently commercially available, most contain surfactants as their active ingredient; such ingredients apparently are spermicidal by virtue of their ability to disrupt the integrity of the sperm cell membrane. These contraceptive products can be demonstrated to immobilize sperm effectively *in vitro*; nevertheless, such effectiveness, demonstrable in the laboratory, cannot necessarily be extrapolated to the actual clinical situation, as evidenced by the fact that both low, as well as high, use effectiveness rates have been reported for them.

A considerable number of plants have been screened *in vitro* for spermicidal activity, and preliminary results reported;[162] the ability of the plant extracts to immobilize rat sperm was investigated first, and those extracts showing activity were then tested against human sperm. Further details concerning the latter extracts and those of other plants, and/or constituents thereof, showing activity against human sperm are presented in Table 3. Unfortunately, virtually no attempts seem to have been made as yet to establish whether or not they might be able to demonstrate similar spermicidal

Table 3. Plants and Plant Constituents Demonstrating Activity Against Human Sperm *In Vitro*.[a]

Plant	Plant Parts	Active Constituents	Reference
Araliaceae			
Schefflera capitata Harms	Aboveground	Scheffleroside (XIX)	162-164
Caryophyllaceae			
Gypsophila cerastioides D. Don	Whole	Saponins	162,163
Combretaceae			
Terminalia bellerica Roxb.	Fruit	Saponins	163
Compositae			
Calendula officinalis L.	Flowers	Total saponins	165
Solidago virgaurea L.	Whole	Saponins	162,163
Gramineae			
Dimeria gracilis Nees ex Steud.	Whole	Saponins	162,163
Labiatae			
Anisomeles malabarica R. Br. ex Sims	Aboveground	Saponins	162,163
Leguminosae			
Aeschynomene indica L.	Whole	Saponins	162,163
Albizia lebbek Benth.[b]	Pod, root	Echinocystic and oleanolic acid glycosides	162,163
Pithecellobium saman Benth.	Flowers	Samanin-D (XX)	166
Pterolobium indicum A. Rich.	Aboveground	Saponins	162,163
Samanea saman Merr.	Aboveground	Saponins	162,163
Trigonella foenum-graecum L.	Seed	Hederagenin glycosides	162,163
Myrsinaceae			
Ardisia neriifolia Wall.	Aboveground	-[c]	162
Phytolaccaceae			
Phytolacca dodecandra L'Herit.	Fruit	Lemmatoxin (XXI)	165

Table 3. Plants and Plant Constituents Demonstrating Activity Against Human Sperm *In Vitro*.[a] (continued).

Plant	Plant Parts	Active Constituents	Reference
Pittosporaceae			
Pittosporum neelgherense Wight & Arnott	Aboveground	-[c]	162
Ranunculaceae			
Caltha palustris L.	Whole	Saponins	162,163
Sapindaceae			
Blighia sapida	Fruit	Hederagenin and oleanolic acid glycosides	163
Sapindus mukorossi Gaertn.	Fruit	Hederagenin glycosides	163
Sapotaceae			
Madhuca butyracea (Roxb.) Macbride	Seed	Bassic acid glycosides	162,163
Madhuca latifolia	Seed	Bassic acid glycosides	163
Verbenaceae			
Clerodendrum serratum (L.) Moon	Aboveground	Saponins	162,163

[a] Specific tests used varied among the studies and included the Spot Test and the International Planned Parenthood Federation (IPPF) Agreed Test.
[b] Lebbekanin-E, a glycoside of acacic acid containing glucose, arabinose, xylose, and rhamnose in a molar ratio of 4:2:1:1, has been isolated from the wood of *A. lebbek* and reported to exhibit spermicidal activity.[167] The species of sperm used and the manner of testing were not indicated.
[c] Activity was reported only for the crude 50% aqueous ethanol extract.

activity in the *in vivo* situation as well.

Solvent fractionation of a 70% aqueous ethanol extract of the aboveground parts of *Schefflera capitata* localized the spermicidal activity in the defatted 1-butanol soluble fraction, from which was isolated a saponin given the name, scheffleroside (XIX);[164] the latter, at a 0.05% concentration, was able to kill human sperm instantaneously in both the Spot and IPPF Agreed Tests. When subjected to acid hydrolysis, scheffleroside yielded one mole each of echinocystic acid, fucose, galactose, and glucuronic acid.

Stolzenberg and Parkhurst[165] investigated the spermicidal activity of (a) the crude saponin fraction from *Calendula officinalis*, *Phytolacca dodecandra*, and *Phytolacca americana*; and (b) three purified saponins [lemmatoxin (XXI), lemmatoxin-C (XXII), and oleanoglycotoxin-A (XXIII)] obtained from *P. dodecandra*. Inhibition of the motility of human sperm was produced *in vitro* by the crude saponin fraction of *P. dodecandra* and *C. officinalis*, and by lemmatoxin. Oleanoglycotoxin-A was only weakly active and the crude saponin preparation from *P. americana* was inactive. Since both purified saponins are trisaccharides of oleanolic acid, the variation in activity between them might be attributable to the types of sugar attached, and to the arrangement of their attachment, to each other and to the aglycone.[165] Lemmatoxin-C, also a trisaccharide of oleanolic acid, was not tested against human sperm, but did show activity against rat sperm *in vitro*.

It is interesting that the *P. americana* saponin fraction, reportedly containing phytolaccagenin as the principal aglycone,[165] failed to show activity against human sperm *in vitro*. Shaaban and Ahmed[168] had earlier reported the isolation of a steroidal saponin from the root of this plant and had stated that its activity correlated in all respects with that reported for the root and its crude extracts. The data they presented indicated that this saponin

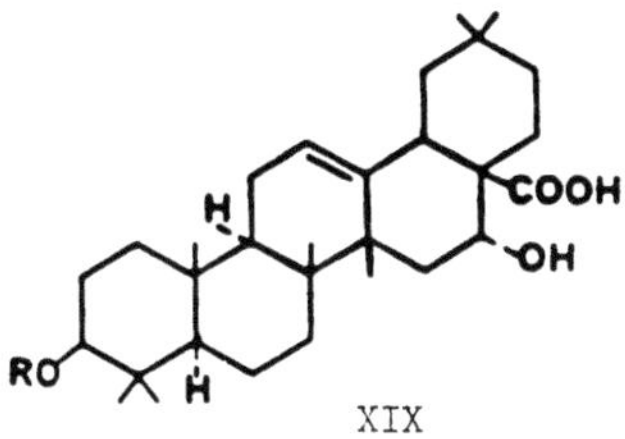

XIX

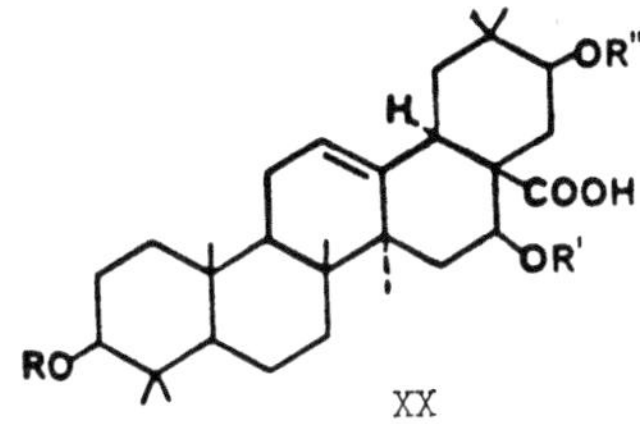

XX

R = Fucose-Galactose-Glucuronic acid-

R - R' - R" = Glucose:Arabinose:
Xylose:Rhamnose
(5:4:3:1)

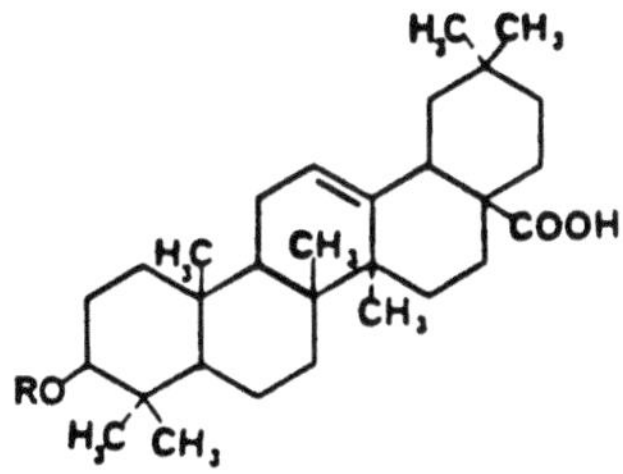

XXI R =

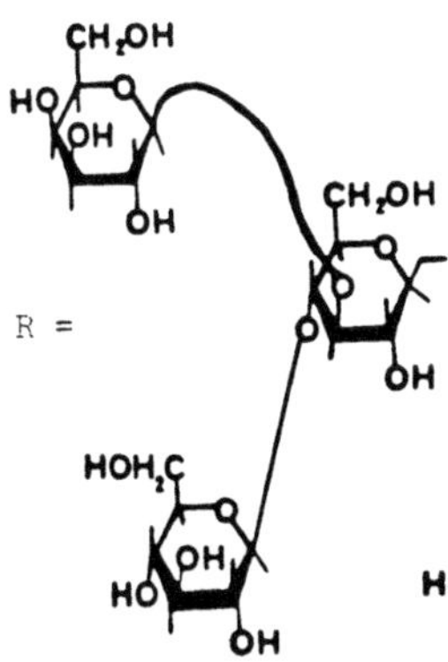

XXII R =

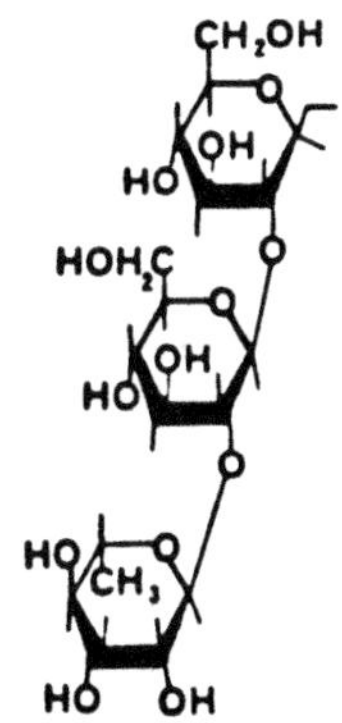

XXIII R =

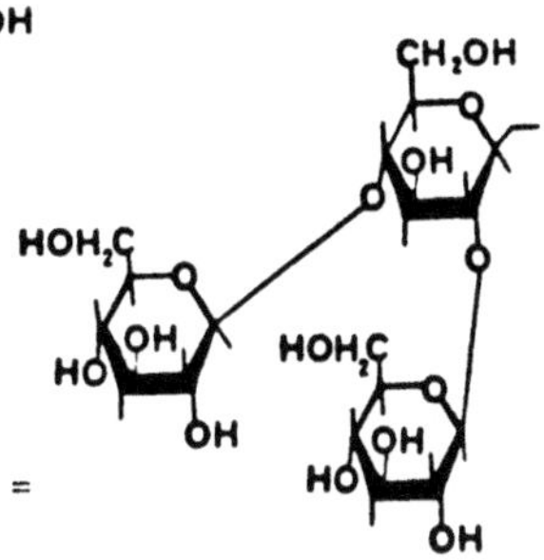

FIG. 4: Plant constituents (XIX-XXIII) reportedly showing activity against human and/or rat sperm *in vitro*.
See text for further details.

was active against human sperm *in vitro*. They also reported contraceptive efficacy for this saponin in a small clinical trial. However, the significance of the latter report is questionable since no data concerning frequency of intercourse, for example, were presented. Furthermore, the aqueous solution of the drug was applied by soaking a piece of cotton in it, and then placing the cotton high in the vagina shortly before intercourse. Whether or not the stated clinical efficacy might have been due to the cotton plug's serving as a mechanical barrier in much the same way as do the investigational intravaginal sponge type contraceptives,[161] is not clear.

Setty *et al.*[163] further fractionated the 50% aqueous ethanol plant extracts previously reported[162] to exhibit activity against human sperm *in vitro*. The spermicidal activity in each case was found to be localized in the 1-butanol soluble fraction of the water soluble/petroleum ether and benzene insoluble fraction of the aqueous ethanol extract, and to be due to the saponins present in that fraction. The results of preliminary testing of the total saponin fraction from *Sapindus mukorossi* fruit, in the form of a vaginally applied cream, reportedly showed a lack of toxicity in both rabbits and rhesus monkeys.[163]

Samanin-D (XX) is yet another saponin which has shown activity against both rat and human sperm in the *in vitro* Spot Test.[166] This compound was obtained by further extraction and fractionation of an ethanol extract of the petroleum ether defatted flowers of *Pitheoellobium saman*. Samanin-D has been partially characterized as a glycoside of acacic acid with 13 moles of four sugars: glucose, arabinose, xylose, and rhamnose, in a molar ratio of 5:4:3:1, respectively.

V. FERTILITY CONTROL IN THE MALE

Compared with the large number of plants reported to be used ethnomedically, or tested experimentally, for fertility control in the female, relatively few have been reported thusly for fertility control in the male.[4] Work has been reported concerning the potential usefulness of employing chemosterilants to control rodent[169] and insect[170] populations; also, impaired fertility may present clinically as a side effect of therapy with antineoplastic[171] and other cytotoxic[172] agents. However, the use of such types of drug, whether natural or synthetic, for purposely controlling fertility in the human male has not yet proven feasible; the ability of antineoplastic agents, for example, to induce chromosomal aberrations,[173] rather than merely suppress sperm count, plus their potential for causing other serious adverse reactions, preclude their use as fertility regulating agents. Nevertheless, as was already pointed out with respect to the possibility of interrupting pregnancy with cytotoxic compounds (*vide supra*), the presence of such constituents in plants might also account for a lack of fertility in males ingesting them.

Inhibition of the spermatogenic function of the testis by the total alkaloid fraction of *Catharanthus roseus* (Apocynaceae),[174] and by its isolated alkaloids, vinblastine[175-177] and vincristine,[177,178] has been studied in the rat[174,176,177] and/or mouse.[175,178] Results included (a) evidence of mitotic and meiotic arrest[177] which may have been due to an induced decrease in cytoplasmic microtubules and an inhibition of centriole migration;[175] (b) impaired spermatogonial differentiation;[176] (c) opening of the cytoplasmic bridges between the spermatids, resulting in giant cell formation;[177] (d) loss of microtubules from the Sertoli cells and disturbance of their mitochondria,[177] thus impairing Sertoli cell function as evidenced by premature sloughing of the late spermatids into the lumen of the tubules; and (e) biochemical evidence that nonproliferating cell types, as well as those that are dividing, may be affected;[178] *i.e.* vincristine caused some inhibition of uridine and *l*-leucine incorporation by early and late spermatids, respectively, as well as inhibition of thymidine incorporation by spermatogonia. Lee and Dixon[178] also carried out a serial mating study with mice to assess the animals' fertility after they had been treated with vincristine. A marked decrease in fertility developed within a week after treatment, likewise indicating that even relatively mature spermatid stages, and possibly spermatozoa, had been affected; furthermore, fertility remained impaired, merely approaching the control rate after about 55 days, thus indicating that spermatocytes, and spermatogonia as well, had been affected. The long lag time before recovery of fertility may have been related to the time required for a critical number of spermatogonia to form, such that the latter could then be able to begin differentiating, and thus eventually repopulate the seminiferous tubules with the more mature stages; the latter hypothesis[176] has been based on data obtained from testicular tissue of rats which had been treated with vinblastine.

Extracts of *Aristolochia indica* L. (Aristolochiaceae),[179] *Hibiscus rosa-sinensis* L. (Malvaceae),[180] *Malvaviscus conzattii* Greenm. (Malvaceae),[181,182] and *Momordica charantia* L. (Cucurbitaceae)[183] have been reported to disrupt spermatogenesis in mice,[179] rats,[180,181] gerbils,[181,183] bats,[182] and/or dogs;[183] in contrast, however, with the studies[175-178] involving the isolated alkaloids of *C. roseus*, the experiments investigating the testicular effects of extracts from these four plants have been of a rather preliminary nature.

In the case of the benzene extract of *H. rosa-sinensis* flowers, administered to rats at a daily dose of 250 mg/kg p.o. for 30, 45, or 60 days, the antispermatogenic effect appears to have been indirect, *i.e.* the result of an inhibition of pituitary gonadotropin secretion.[180] Although an *additional* action directly on the testis was not ruled out, evidence was discussed which suggested a central mechanism of action; specifically, histological examination reportedly revealed degranulated pituitary gonadotrophs, while assay results reportedly indicated a decrease in total pituitary gonadotropin content. Decreased seminal vesicle and prostate gland weights, furthermore, indicated a lack of stimulation by testicular androgen, lack of the latter resulting from the presumed decrease in pituitary gonadotropin secretion.

Whereas bioassay results reportedly indicated that this benzene extract did not have androgenic or antiandrogenic activity,[180] both the benzene and alcohol extracts of *H. rosa-sinensis* have been shown to be antiestrogenic.[65] Since the nature of this antiestrogenic activity is unknown,[70] it seems unwise to speculate as to whether it might be responsible for the effects seen in the male. Nevertheless, it may be of interest to note that various synthetic compounds possessing antiestrogenic activity have also been shown to be antispermatogenic in rats, the latter effect apparently resulting from an inhibition of pituitary gonadotropin secretion.[29]

Neither fertility, nor willingness to mate were ascertained in the male rats treated with the extract of *H. rosa-sinensis*; however, the apparent inhibition of androgen secretion,[180] and the detrimental effect that androgen lack may be expected to have on libido, make questionable the practicality of using this plant extract for contraception in the male.

Too few definitive data were reported concerning the effects of the extracts of the other three plants[179,181-183] to indicate with any certainty whether the disruption of spermatogenesis reported with each might have been direct or indirect. Again, neither the fertility of the treated animals, nor their willingness to mate, was determined.

Antifertility effectiveness, yet maintenance of libido and sexual potency, are important criteria that need to be met if an agent is to prove practical for controlling fertility in the male. Histological evidence of spermatogenic arrest and/or the finding of a low sperm count in the ejaculate infer, but do not prove, that agents causing such effects will significantly impair fertility. Despite the histological and biochemical evidence of impaired fertility obtained by Lee and Dixon,[178] for example, the fertility of their mice was not reduced to zero. In the case of the human, if the sperm count is *above* the level of 20 million/ml, there appears to be no correlation between the actual sperm count and the ease of conception;[184] *below* the level of 20 million/ml, however, the proportion of conceptions within any given period of time is lower. Interestingly, it was reported that of 386 men, all of whom had previously fathered at least one child, 20% had sperm counts of less than 20 million/ml at the time of undergoing elective vasectomy for fertility control.[185] Furthermore, Barfield *et al.*[186] recently reviewed their own data, and those of others, which indicated that conceptions had been achieved, albeit at progressively lower rates, by men whose sperm counts apparently were below 20 million/ml, below 10 million/ml, below 5 million/ml, and even below 1 million/ml; such observations suggest, therefore, that a male contraceptive method based on suppression of spermatogenesis would seem to require an end point of sustained azoospermia, if 100% effectiveness were to be the goal. Lack of proof of paternity, of course, must be considered, as well as the point that a sperm count determined at some time before or after the actual time of impregnation may or may not reflect the sperm concentration at the time of impregnation.[186] Furthermore, other factors besides sperm count seem to contribute importantly to the ease of conception, namely (a) percentage of active sperm, (b) quality of their motility, and (c) the frequency of intercourse;[184] none of these factors, of course, are reflected in a sperm count *per se*.

Such points need to be considered when one is evaluating the significance of reports that plant extracts and/or compounds isolated therefrom, have shown fertility regulating effects in the male. In 1958-1959, Sanyal,[187] and Sanyal and Rana,[188] presented preliminary results obtained in human males treated with *m*-xylohydroquinone (XXIV), a compound reportedly isolated from the oil extracted from the seeds of *Pisum sativum* L. (Leguminosae).[189] Control sperm counts were determined on ejaculates from 15 volunteers; four days later, the men were administered *m*-xylohydroquinone, 500-600 mg p.o. A further 24 hours later, a second sperm count was made, and a third count, four days after that. For most of the men, the 24 hour posttreatment ejaculate contained the lowest sperm concentration of the three specimens;[187] however, the lowest 24 hour posttreatment value obtained was 22 million/ml and the highest, 165.5 million/ml. Furthermore, the men with the higher pretreatment sperm counts also tended to have the higher 24 hour and higher four day posttreatment counts while those with the lower initial counts similarly tended to have the lower posttreatment counts. Since (a) variability in sperm counts is a normal occurrence,[186] (b) errors are inherent in performing sperm counts,[185] and (c) none of the sperm counts was below 20 million/ml,[187] the significance of Sanyal's observations to fertility regulation is questionable.

Nevertheless, Sanyal and Rana[188] subsequently administered *m*-xylohydroquinone, 600-700 mg p.o. every two weeks, to 64 men for the purpose of contraception. A reduction in pregnancy rate among the men's wives was reported, compared with the pretreatment pregnancy rate; however, it should be noted that all failures occurred within the first six months of treatment. Perhaps, at best, *m*-xylohydroquinone might have been contraceptive only to those men whose fertility had already spontaneously approached the subnormal level. It should be noted also that the frequency of intercourse was not reported.

Gossypol (XXV), obtained from the seed, stem, and root of *Gossypium hir-*

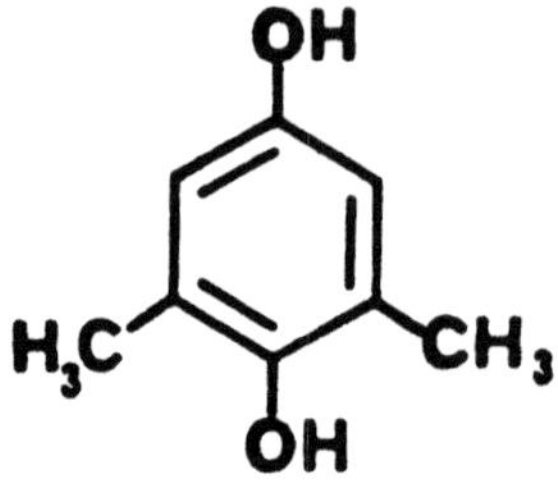

XXIV

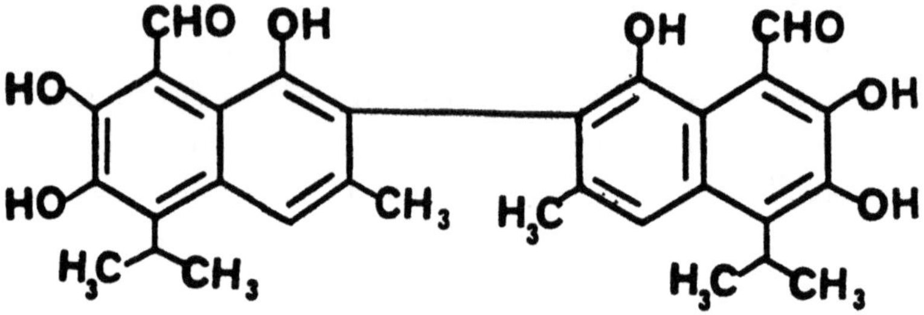

XXV

FIG. 5: Plant constituents (XXIV, XXV) reported to have antifertility effects in the male.

sutum (Malvaceae), and other *Gossypium* species, has been widely publicized as a contraceptive agent effective in 99.89% of 4,000 human males in which it was tested.[190] Careful examination of the original paper,[191] however, reveals that the 99.89% antifertility efficacy value was based on the results of semen analysis; specifically, efficacy was defined as the induction of necrospermia or a sperm count below 4 million/ml, one or the other of these effects apparently being achieved in 99.89% of the subjects. Induction of infertility, thusly defined, usually was accomplished after two months of therapy with gossypol, 20 mg daily, although sometimes more prolonged therapy was required. When "efficacy" had been achieved, the dosage was reduced to a maintenance level of 150-220 mg per month given in divided doses. No data have been reported on pregnancy rate among the partner(s) of men treated with gossypol; furthermore, the only evidence even suggesting that actual contraceptive effectiveness might have been studied are statements that about 6% of the subjects complained of some decrease in libido, but that drug administration was nevertheless able to be continued since potency was not impaired.[191]

Even the published data[191] concerning the antifertility activity of gossypol in lower animals, specifically rats, rabbits, and monkeys, apparently are based on histological evidence, not on the results of mating studies; one minor exception is a statement that gossypol treated male rats sired grossly normal litters when they "were allowed to mate with untreated females after recovery from the antifertility effect of gossypol." Nevertheless, since gossypol currently appears to represent the most promising natural product contraceptive for use in the male, a summary here of the published findings[191] seems warranted.

Histological examination of testicular and epididymal tissues of rats which had been treated with gossypol or gossypol acetic acid at daily doses of

15-40 mg/kg p.o. for two to four weeks revealed damage first to the spermatids and then to the spermatocytes. Desquamation of the germinal epithelium occurred in the form of multinucleated giant cells derived from spermatids and spermatocytes; only Sertoli cells and spermatogonia remained in the seminiferous tubules. Necrotic spermatozoa were found, and the sperm count gradually decreased until an azoospermic level was reached. Desquamated mono-, bi-, and multinucleated spermatids and spermatocytes, as well as malformed spermatozoa, could also be found in the semen of human males treated with gossypol, and apparently azoospermia could be achieved.

Results of chromosome studies reportedly showed no significant difference between the incidence of polyploid cells among the spermatogonia from gossypol treated rats and that among the spermatogonia from control rats. Studies of leukocyte chromosomes from 16 gossypol treated humans and 12 controls also reportedly failed to demonstrate significant differences in the incidence of aberrations and abnormal cells. de Peyster and Wang,[190] furthermore, tested gossypol in the Ames *Salmonella*/mammalian microsome mutagenicity test; the results of two separate assays indicated that gossypol was not mutagenic to the five standard tester strains of *S. typhimurium*, whether or not a rat liver metabolic enzyme fraction had been included.

There also reportedly were no significant differences between controls and gossypol treated rats with respect either to serum luteinizing hormone (LH) levels or to the ultrastructure of the interstitial cells of Leydig.[191] Curiously, the libido of the rats *seemed to be* unaffected. Circulating testosterone and LH levels apparently remained normal in gossypol treated humans.

Certainly, data indicating a contraceptive effect for gossypol, as determined by pregnancy rate among partner(s) of treated men, would be welcome. However, further studies concerning possible toxicity also seem warranted.

Gossypol is a lipid soluble compound,[190] shown experimentally to be eliminated from the body rather slowly;[191] thus, the potential for *accumulated* toxicity should be considered. Toxic effects were not reported in rats treated with doses of gossypol adequate to disrupt spermatogenesis.[191] Clinically, the chief side effect reportedly was transient weakness occurring early in therapy. The relationship, if any, between gossypol ingestion on the one hand, and, on the other, the hypokalemia, mild electrocardiographic changes, and transient elevations in serum glutamic pyruvic transaminase level reported for some patients, remains to be determined. Prolonged high dosing with gossypol or with its source, cottonseed meal, has been shown to be lethal to swine, evidence of toxicity being found in the heart, liver, and kidneys;[192] lung edema and variable degrees of inflammation in the gastrointestinal tract were also observed. Whether or not the reported selective toxicity of low doses of gossypol on the seminiferous tubules[191] can be substantiated and employed as a practical method of fertility control in the male, awaits further investigation.

VI. DISCUSSION

This review began by stating that since many other types of pharmacologically active agent have been found in the plant kingdom, it was logical to presume that fertility regulating agents might also be found there. Certainly, we have presented a few examples supportive of this presumption, although their *practical* application to fertility control in the human remains to be demonstrated. Since voluminous folklore[2,3,4] and suggestive, albeit inadequate experimental results[2,3,4] would lead one to believe that useful fertility regulating agents do exist in plants, one is forced to ask why, if that is so, have they continued to elude investigators. There are many possible explanations.

From an ecologic point of view, it would seem unlikely that a great many plant species could be discovered which would consistently contain readily ingestible quantities of agents extremely effective in inhibiting fertility in numerous animal species. The following represent more logical explanations, from the point of view of maintaining the balance of nature. (a) The content of fertility regulating compound(s) in a given species may vary in relation to some environmental factor(s). (b) Fertility regulating compounds may be present in a given species but may possess such weak activity that only the most sensitive and/or already subfertile humans or other animals may respond. (c) A number of fertility regulating compounds, having either similar or different mechanisms of action, may be present in a given species, but all the compounds may possess relatively weak activity; when the plant is tested experimentally, fertility regulating activity may not be demonstrable because the active components may have been separated due to extraction/fractionation procedures and/or because not all of the types of activity present, which types may have to work in conjunction to impair fertility, may be demonstrable in the test system(s) chosen. Another possibility is that the nature of the active constituent(s) of a given species may be such that fertility reduction will be achieved only if both male and female partners are treated; *i.e.* the constituent(s) may at best be capable of producing subnormal fertility, but not infertility, in either male or female alone. A still further possibility with respect to crude extracts or only semipurified fractions is that toxic constituents may be present as well as fertility regulating ones; it may have been assumed, however, that the toxic and antifertility effects observed were due to the *same* constituent(s) and therefore, the possibility of separating such activities may have remained unexplored. Admittedly, these ideas are rather speculative, but some illustrative examples will be cited (A. Plant factors) which provide some rational basis for such speculations.

Other answers as to why fertility regulating agents have eluded investigators may lie with the investigators themselves. These will be discussed under B. Investigator factors.

Thirdly, much of the belief that fertility regulating agents of some sort do exist in the plant kingdom is based on ethnomedical (folkloric) reports. While we do feel that folklore is a justifiable basis, at least on which to begin selecting plants to be tested experimentally for fertility regulating activity, we must nevertheless consider that variability may exist among cultures with respect to their "definitions" of fertility, infertility, and contraceptive efficacy. The connotation of contraceptive efficacy today, in the era of the almost 100% effective combination type oral hormonal contraceptives,[10,11] cannot be the same as it was before their advent. Such points will be considered further under C. Observer factors.

A. Plant factors

To begin with, it seems reasonable that various factors (*e.g.* soil, climate, other geographic phenomena, and perhaps genetics) reportedly capable of influencing the phytochemical content of plants in general,[193,194] may likewise influence the content of fertility regulating principle(s) of plants reputedly possessing such activity. More specifically, with respect to estrogenic plants, the phytoestrogen content of *Medicago sativa* (Leguminosae), *Glycine max*, and *Trifolium repens* has been reported to increase in response to fungal disease.[14]

Fungal disease of other plants may also be of significance with respect to fertility regulation, but in the examples to be cited, products of the fungi themselves, rather than products induced to be synthesized by the plants, appear to be the compounds of interest. The classic example, of course, concerns the infection of rye [*Secale cereale* (Gramineae)] by the fungus, *Claviceps purpurea*.[118] As already discussed (*vide supra*), abortion was a frequent complication of ergot poisoning resulting from consumption of contaminated grain.

Fusarium roseum is a fungus which infects corn [*Zea mays* (Gramineae)] and other grains, and produces an estrogenic mycotoxin, zearalenone, under certain environmental conditions.[195] Ingestion of zearalenone by sows reportedly is associated with a syndrome including the appearance of external signs of estrus, and a decreased ovulation rate. Its effects, if any, on mature boars are still being investigated;[195] however, it has been reported that young boars ingesting zearalenone contaminated grain, may develop testicular atrophy and mammary gland enlargement.[196]

In 1972, Chow *et al.*[197] reported the disruption of pregnancy in mice fed an aqueous fraction of pine [*Pinus ponderosa* (Pinaceae)] needles, but similar fractions of needles harvested during the following two years appeared to be devoid of activity.[198] Fractions tested following their incubation with fungi which had previously been observed on the pine needles, did produce pregnancy disruption. The authors concluded that the effects they had reported earlier[197] had probably not been due to constituents of the pine needles, but rather to mycotoxins which may have been produced by fungi contaminating the pine needles.[198] A syndrome, pine needle "abortion," has been reported to occur in cattle ingesting *P. ponderosa* needles during the last trimester of pregnancy.[199] The syndrome actually is characterized by weak uterine contractions, excessive uterine hemorrhage, incomplete cervical dilatation, birth of a calf which may survive, and a retained placenta. Whether the syndrome seen in cattle is due to normal chemical constituents of the pine needles themselves, or to mycotoxins, remains to be determined. Considering the observations which have been made in mice[197,198] and cattle,[199] it is interesting to note that Indian women of Washington,[199] Oregon,[199] and Colorado[197] reportedly drank aqueous extracts of *P. ponderosa* needles for the purpose of inducing abortion.

Regarding the possibility that fertility regulating substances may be present in plants, yet be of too weak activity to affect most individuals, we can cite a case report of a previously fertile patient who developed azoospermia in response to colchicine (*Colchicum* sp.) therapy.[172] The patient's sperm count returned to normal, and his fertility returned, after colchicine was discontinued, but he again became azoospermic after colchicine therapy (0.01 grain b.i.d.) was reinstituted. It seems likely that azoospermia in this patient did result from colchicine therapy, but it probably represents a rare side effect in a sensitive patient. Bremner and Paulsen[200] subsequently studied the effect on sperm count and hormone levels, of 1.8-2.4 mg colchicine administered daily for several months to a small number of men; their results, as well as other published evidence they cited, suggest that colchicine does *not* commonly lower sperm counts or impair fertility.

Concerning the presence of multiple active compounds in a plant, we can first cite a study[201] in which an extract of *Trifolium repens* was reported to possess an estrogenic activity equivalent to that of 480 mcg coumestrol/g. When the extract was separated into five fractions on a silica gel column, two of the five fractions were each found to possess an estrogenic activity equivalent to about only 120 mcg coumestrol/g. Bioassay of a recombined aliquot of these two fractions gave a value of 416 mcg coumestrol/g. The authors speculated that one of these fractions may have contained coumestrol and the other, another estrogenically active coumestan, repensol. By means of a uterine weight bioassay, the presence of estrogenic activity in the two fractions could still be demonstrated even though the level of activity of each was only half that of the original fraction. In contrast, if an entire extract of some plant possessed antiovulatory, antiimplantation, or abortifacient activity, due to the cumulative activity of a number of compounds, separation of such an extract might yield fractions possessing activity too weak to be demonstrable in a bioassay in which an *event*, rather than a weight change measureable in mg, was the endpoint.

As already discussed (*vide supra*), *Montanoa tomentosa* contains two uterine stimulants, zoapatanol and montanol, the former apparently being the more potent of the two when tested *in situ*;[145] zoapatanol was also reported capable of interrupting pregnancy in the guinea pig in a dosage range of 25-85 mg/kg. One wonders, however, whether administering the weaker montanol simultaneously with zoapatanol might yield even better results; certainly, the ethnomedical preparation of *M. tomentosa*, reputed to be used as an abortifacient,[145] contains both compounds.

Although no well documented examples may be cited at this time, it is interesting to note that if a plant possessed weak cytotoxic activity, it might impair, but not totally eliminate an implanting embryo. However, if the plant also contained a weak uterine stimulant, the *added* effect of this compound might nevertheless serve to terminate the pregnancy. If this plant were tested for only a short period during pregnancy, its overall fertility regulating activity might not be demonstrable.

The potential, yet impractical, fertility regulating activity of cytotoxic antineoplastic agents has been discussed (*vide supra*) in relation both to pregnancy interruption and to inhibition of spermatogenesis. Apparently, such agents may also sometimes impair ovarian follicular development and possibly even destroy oocytes.[173] It thus seems reasonable to speculate that weakly active cytotoxic compounds might be present in a plant; that an occasional male, such as the one cited earlier,[172] might respond to its usage with a decreased sperm count, apparently in the absence of other side effects; and that simultaneous usage of this plant by his partner might at least temporarily suppress her ovarian function. The assumption is being made that other toxic effects will not be manifested in the couple. Hence, the activity and/or concentration of the cytotoxic compound(s) may be too low to demonstrate activity in the laboratory unless *pairs* of animals are treated and tested for fertility. However, one should not rule out the possibility of discovering phytochemicals which might prove to be *selectively* cytotoxic to some component(s) of the reproductive system.

B. Investigator factors

Lack of correlation may be found in the literature[4] between experimental results obtained by different investigators, between those obtained *in vitro* and *in vivo*, and between experimental results and information found in folklore. The contributory effect of inadequate numbers of vehicle treated controls has already been commented upon (*vide supra*) as has that of variability in the plants themselves (A. Plant factors). Other contributory factors relating to screening of plants for pharmacologic activity in general,[1] and for fertility regulating activity in particular,[3,202] have also been discussed previously. Of particular significance may be the difficulties involved in testing extracts which may be insoluble, or only barely soluble, in commonly employed, nontoxic diluents;[1] and the diversity in reproductive function and control thereof, among various laboratory species, as well as in comparison with the human.[2,202] That plants may not have been properly identified is an additional explanation. The importance of documenting plant collections, and even ethnomedical reports if possible, with a voucher specimen,[1] and of identifying a plant not only by genus and species, and by cultivar if applicable, but also by the name(s) of the authority for the taxon,[5] cannot be overemphasized. It should be noted that a number of the references cited in this chapter did not contain authority citations for the plants reported on therein.

C. Observer factors

Interpreting the significance of folkloric reports that a plant is contraceptive and/or abortifacient may be the greatest problem, particularly since one may be unaware as to what was considered a normal and/or desirable fertility rate in that culture, at the time the plant was thusly designated; likewise, the influence that various sexual practices and/or taboos might have had on fertility rate may be unknown. On the other hand, that use of the same plant for the same purpose by different peoples lends credence to its possible effectiveness, was commented on earlier (*vide supra*).

Price,[203] nevertheless has pointed out the difficulty in establishing a cause and effect relationship between the use of certain plants and the absence of evidence of pregnancy, *versus* establishing such a relationship between the use of certain plants and the alleviation of some ailment. Assuming the disease being treated is not one which readily resolves spontaneously, the use of a given plant, followed most of the time by remission of the disease, tends to suggest that the plant does indeed contain a therapeutically active principle(s). However, the time interval between the use of a given plant and the appearance, or lack thereof, of evidence of pregnancy is so long, and the causes of relative (or absolute) infertility so numerous,[185] that crediting a plant with contraceptive (or sterilizing) properties, in the absence of scientific experimentation, would appear to be unsound.

For "contraception" to be more than merely coincidental to the use of a plant would seem to imply, furthermore, that the plant is being used at a time during which some antifertility mechanism can operate. Even if one considers all the possible sites and mechanisms for contraceptive action,[2] it is difficult to speculate how the flowers of *Sesbania aegyptiaca* Poir. (Leguminosae), for example, taken for three days *during* menstruation,[204] might be able to inhibit conception, unless, of course, the active principle(s) had a very long duration of action. That such a possibility would not seem applicable, at least not to an Ayurvedic preparation (coded ROC 101), containing other botanicals, is suggested by the report that a preliminary clinical trial with the latter preparation, given for four days *during menstruation*, had to be discontinued because of many *accidental* pregnancies.[205] One must wonder, therefore, particularly, although not exclusively, with respect to folkloric reports, whether individuals attributing contraceptive efficacy, or lack thereof, to plants, have a sufficiently adequate knowledge of reproductive phenomena such that they can draw reasonable conclusions.

Even with respect to plants supposedly possessing abortifacient activity, a cause and effect relationship, in the absence of scientific experimentation, again may only be surmised since abortion can occur spontaneously, most likely before the sixteenth week of gestation, but possibly as late as the twenty-eighth week;[123] after that time, moreover, the chance of spontaneous *delivery* gradually increases from 1:625 at 28 weeks to 1:3.5 at 40 weeks.[206]

Folkloric reports in themselves, therefore, may merely reflect coincidental occurrences; whether various infertility mechanisms might be contributing to the phenomena is probably unknown to the observers, and consequently not reported. Furthermore, the relative proportion of times that use of given plants is followed by lack of pregnancy, or by occurrence of abortion, *versus* the relative proportion of times that such effects do not follow their usage, also is not readily apparent in these reports. Folkloric reports concerning

fertil

lated case reports concerning some interesting, unexpected, useful, peculiar, harmful, *etc.* effect observed in a patient being treated with a commercially available drug. Such an observation in itself does not imply that all patients will respond similarly. However, if sufficient numbers of reports appear from different sources, concerning different patients, it becomes more likely that the relationship is a causal one, even if the response does not occur in all patients. For example, isolated case reports concerning thromboembolic complications in women using oral hormonal contraceptives first began to appear in 1961;[8] numerous similar case reports continued to appear, and a number of retrospective and prospective studies were undertaken to ascertain whether the association between oral contraceptive use and increased risk of circulatory system disease, suggested by the case reports, were real. Only recently,[6] however, after much investigation, has the actual magnitude of the risk become somewhat clear, as well as the degree to which other factors, *e.g.* age and smoking, may contribute to the risk.

D. Conclusions

Ethnomedical reports concerning fertility regulating plants likewise have served to stimulate basic and clinical research aimed at isolating and identifying the active principle(s). Despite some promising leads, however, definitive data are not available, due, we feel, to problems such as those discussed above, and not to an actual absence of orally active plant constituents which could be used safely for fertility regulation in males and/or females.

Drug development programs which involve the *synthesis* of useful compounds are complex, requiring intensive effort by organized teams of highly qualified investigators. Even so, it might take 10 years to produce a safe, effective agent ready for evaluation in the human. Furthermore, not all compounds that enter clinical trials, emerge as marketable drugs. It thus seems logical to expect that similar high intensity programs, well organized and appropriately budgeted, would have to be implemented if useful fertility regulating agents are to be isolated from plants and identified. Only recently, however, has such a program[5] been undertaken.

Specifically, in 1976, the Special Programme of Research, Development, and Research Training in Human Reproduction of the World Health Organization, initiated a comprehensive program designed to discover from plants, fertility regulating agents which would be safe and orally active in humans. The program, which is the responsibility of a unit designated as the Task Force on Indigenous Plants for Fertility Regulation, is a multidisciplinary, multi-centered collaborative one, involving cooperating groups in England, Brazil, Sri Lanka, Hong Kong, South Korea, and the United States. Central to the program is the comprehensive, ongoing accumulation and evaluation of literature concerning plants alleged to have one or more types of ethnopharmacologic use and/or experimentally determined pharmacologic activity, relating to fertility regulation. Data are weighted and analyzed by computer, thus producing rank ordered lists of "priority" plants to be investigated further in these six centers. Of particular interest to the program are leads concerning plants which may interfere with implantation in the female, and those which may interfere with sperm formation and/or maturation in the male.

This multidisciplinary approach, *i.e.* the cooperative participation of pharmacologists, reproductive physiologists, chemists, and botanists, together with input from statisticians, is designed to avoid many of the types of problem we have been discussing. Also, considering the varied types of expertise involved in this program, adequate follow-up of any preliminary interesting data obtained should be possible; such follow-up often appears to be lacking regarding much of the published[4] basic research concerning reputed fertility regulating plants. In time, we will learn whether this multicentered program will indeed have achieved the goals that small scale programs obviously have not achieved to date.

ACKNOWLEDGMENTS

Collection, compilation, and computerization of the literature cited has been supported, in part, through funds from the World Health Organization, Special Programme of Research, Development, and Research Training in Human Reproduction (Project 78135), and from the National Cancer Institute (U.S.A.) (contract CM-97259).

The authors also wish to thank Mr. Chun-Tao Che for translating into English, much of the work which has been published in Chinese, concerning trichosanthin.

REFERENCES

1. Farnsworth, N.R., and Bingel, A.S., Problems and prospects of discovering new drugs from higher plants by pharmacological screening, in *New Natural Products and Plant Drugs with Pharmacological, Biological, or Therapeutical Activity*, Wagner, H., and Wolff, P., Eds., Springer-Verlag, Berlin, 1977, 1.

2. Farnsworth, N.R., Bingel, A.S., Cordell, G.A., Crane, F.A., and Fong, H.H.S., Potential value of plants as sources of new antifertility agents I, *J. Pharm. Sci.*, 64, 535, 1975.

3. Farnsworth, N.R., Bingel, A.S., Cordell, G.A., Crane, F.A., and Fong, H.H.S., Potential value of plants as sources of new antifertility agents II, *J. Pharm. Sci.*, 64, 717, 1975.

4. NAPRALERT (A computer-based natural product data retrieval system) Department of Pharmacognosy and Pharmacology, College of Pharmacy, University of Illinois at the Medical Center, Chicago, Illinois, August 29, 1979.

5. Soejarto, D.D., Bingel, A.S., Slaytor, M., and Farnsworth, N.R., Fertility regulating agents from plants, *Bull. WHO*, 56, 343, 1978.

6. Rinehart, W., and Piotrow, P.T., OCs - update on usage, safety, and side effects, *Pop. Rep.*, Series A, 133, 1979.

7. Lednicer, D., and Mitscher, L.A., *The Organic Chemistry of Drug Synthesis*, John Wiley and Sons, New York, 1977, chap. 10.

8. Bingel, A.S., and Benoit, P.S., Oral contraceptives: therapeutics *versus* adverse reactions, with an outlook for the future I, *J. Pharm. Sci.*, 62, 179, 1973.

9. Bingel, A.S., and Benoit, P.S., Oral contraceptives: therapeutics *versus* adverse reactions, with an outlook for the future II, *J. Pharm. Sci.*, 62, 349, 1973.

10. Henzl, M.R., Natural and synthetic female sex hormones, in *Reproductive Endocrinology: Physiology, Pathophysiology, and Clinical Management*, Yen, S.S.C., and Jaffe, R.B., Eds., W.B. Saunders Co., Philadelphia, 1978, chap. 20.

11. Speroff, L., Glass, R.H., and Kase, N.G., *Clinical Gynecologic Endocrinology and Infertility*, 2nd ed., The Williams & Wilkins Co., Baltimore, 1978, chap. 14.

12. Rudel, H.W., and Kincl, F.A., The biology of anti-fertility steroids, *Acta Endocrinol. Suppl.*, 105, 7, 1966.

13. Rinehart, W., Postcoital contraception - an appraisal, *Pop. Rep.*, Series J, 141, 1976.

14. Livingston, A.L., Forage plant estrogens, *J. Toxicol. Environ. Health*, 4, 301, 1978.

15. Adams, N.R., Morphological changes in the organs of ewes grazing oestrogenic subterranean clover, *Res. Vet. Sci.*, 22, 216, 1977.

16. Findlay, J.K., Buckmaster, J.M., Chamley, W.A., Cumming, I.A., Hearnshaw, H., and Goding, J.R., Release of luteinizing hormone by oestradiol-17β and a gonadotrophin-releasing hormone in ewes affected with clover disease, *Neuroendocrinology*, 11, 57, 1973.

17. Lightfoot, R.J., Croker, K.P., and Neil, H.G., Failure of sperm transport in relation to ewe infertility following prolonged grazing on oestrogenic pastures, *Aust. J. Agr. Res.*, 18, 755, 1967.

18. Mattner, P.E., Formation and retention of the spermatozoan reservoir in the cervix of the ruminant, *Nature* (London), 212, 1479, 1966.

19. Smith, J.F., Studies on ovine infertility in agricultural regions of western Australia: cervical mucus production by fertile and infertile ewes, *Aust. J. Agr. Res.*, 22, 513, 1971.

20. Adams, N.R., Cervical mucus changes in infertile ewes previously exposed to oestrogenic subterranean clover, *Res. Vet. Sci.*, 21, 59, 1976.

21. Shutt, D.A., The effects of plant oestrogens on animal reproduction, *Endeavour*, 35, 110, 1976.

22. Biggers, J.D., Plant phenols possessing oestrogenic activity, in *The Pharmacology of Plant Phenolics*, Fairbairn, J.W., Ed., Academic Press, New York, 1959, 51.

23. Shemesh, M., Lindner, H.R., and Ayalon, N., Affinity of rabbit uterine oestradiol receptor for phyto-oestrogens and its use in a competitive protein-binding radioassay for plasma coumestrol, *J. Reprod. Fert.*, 29, 1, 1972.

24. Shutt, D.A., and Cox, R.I., Steroid and phyto-oestrogen binding to sheep uterine receptors *in vitro*, *J. Endocrinol.*, 52, 299, 1972.

25. Folman, Y., and Pope, G.S., The interaction in the immature mouse of potent oestrogens with coumestrol, genistein, and other utero-vaginotrophic compounds of low potency, *J. Endocrinol.*, 34, 215, 1966.

26. Folman, Y., and Pope, G.S., Effect of norethisterone acetate, dimethylstilboestrol, genistein, and coumestrol on uptake of [^{3}H]oestradiol by uterus, vagina, and skeletal muscle of immature mice, *J. Endocrinol.*, 44, 213, 1969.

27. Martin, P.M., Horwitz, K.B., Ryan, D.S., and McGuire, W.L., Phytoestrogen interaction with estrogen receptors in human breast cancer cells, *Endocrinology*, 103, 1860, 1978.

28. Speroff, L., Glass, R.H., and Kase, N.G., *Clinical Gynecologic Endocrinology and Infertility*, 2nd ed., The Williams & Wilkins Co., Baltimore, 1978, chap. 1.

29. Jackson, H., Antispermatogenic agents, *Brit. Med. Bull.*, 26, 79, 1970.

30. Bounds, D.G., and Pope, G.S., Light-absorption and chemical properties of miroestrol, the oestrogenic substance of *Pueraria mirifica*, *J. Chem. Soc.*, 1960, 3696, 1960.

31. Jones, H.E.H., and Pope, G.S., A study of the action of miroestrol and other oestrogens on the reproductive tract of the immature female mouse, *J. Endocrinol.*, 20, 229, 1960.

32. Terenius, L., Structural characteristics of oestrogen binding in the mouse uterus: inhibition of 17β-oestradiol binding *in vitro* by a plant oestrogen, miroestrol, *Acta Pharmacol. Toxicol.*, 26, 15, 1968.

33. Taylor, N.E., Hodgkin, D.C., and Rollett, J.S., The x-ray crystallographic determination of the structure of bromomiroestrol, *J. Chem. Soc.*, 1960, 3685, 1960.

34. Cain, J.C., Miroestrol: an oestrogen from the plant *Pueraria mirifica*, *Nature* (London), 188, 774, 1960.

35. Jones, H.E.H., and Pope, G.S., A method for the isolation of miroestrol from *Pueraria mirifica*, *J. Endocrinol.*, 22, 303, 1961.

36. Anonymous, An antifertility drug from ethnobotany folklore, in *Regional Research Laboratory News Letter*, Vol. 6, Kapur, B.M., Ed., C.K. Atal, Publisher, Jammu-Tawi, 1979, 6.

37. Bhutani, S.P., Chibber, S.S., and Seshadri, T.R., Components of the roots of *Pueraria tuberosa*: isolation of a new isoflavone-*C*-glycoside (Di-*O*-acetylpuerarin), *Indian J. Chem.*, 7, 210, 1969.

38. Speroff, L., Glass, R.H., and Kase, N.G., *Clinical Gynecologic Endocrinology and Infertility*, 2nd ed., The Williams & Wilkins Co., Baltimore, 1978, chap. 9.

39. *Stedman's Medical Dictionary*, 22nd ed., The Williams & Wilkins Co., Baltimore, 1972, 276.

40. Kaymakcalan, S., and Topuz, Ü., The effect of morphine addiction on the oestrous cycle in rats, *Acta Med.*, 7, 49, 1970.

41. Libertun, C., and McCann, S.M., Blockade of the release of gonadotropins and prolactin by subcutaneous or intraventricular injection of atropine in male and female rats, *Endocrinology*, 92, 1714, 1973.

42. Khanna, U., and Chaudhury, R.R., Rapid screening of possible antiovulatory substances using copper-induced ovulation in rabbits, *Indian J. Pharm.*, 30, 148, 1968.

43. Dorfman, R.I., Hormonal contraception, *Life Sci.*, 14, 827, 1974.

44. Morris, J.M., and van Wagenen, G., Interception: the use of postovulatory estrogens to prevent implantation, *Amer. J. Obstet. Gynecol.*, 115, 101, 1973.

45. Sparrow, M.J., Oestrogen interception: the morning-after pill, *N. Z. Med. J.*, 79, 862, 1974.

46. Haspels, A.A., Interception: post-coital estrogens in 3016 women, *Contraception*, 14, 375, 1976.

47. Naqvi, R.H., and Warren, J.C., Interceptives: drugs interrupting pregnancy after implantation, *Steroids*, 18, 731, 1971.

48. Pakrashi, A., Chakrabarty, B., and Dasgupta, A., Effects of the extracts from *Aristolochia indica* Linn. on interception in female mice, *Experientia*, 32, 394, 1976.

49. Pakrashi, A., and Chakrabarty, B., Biological properties of interceptive agents from *Aristolochia indica* Linn., *Indian J. Med. Res.*, 66, 991, 1977.

50. Pakrashi, A., and Shaha, C., Effect of a sesquiterpene from *Aristolochia indica* Linn. on fertility in female mice, *Experientia*, 33, 1498, 1977.

51. Pakrashi, A., and Pakrasi, P., Biological profile of *p*-coumaric acid

isolated from *Aristolochia indica* Linn., *Indian J. Exp. Biol.*, 16, 1285, 1978.

52. Pakrashi, A., and Pakrasi, P., Antifertility efficacy of the plant *Aristolochia indica* Linn. on mouse, *Contraception*, 20, 49, 1979.

53. Pakrashi, A., and Shaha, C., Effect of methyl ester of aristolic acid from *Aristolochia indica* Linn. on fertility of female mice, *Experientia*, 34, 1192, 1978.

54. Pakrashi, A., and Pakrasi, P.L., Interceptive and abortifacient activity of *Aristolochia indica* L. and possible mode of action, *Indian J. Exp. Biol.*, 15, 428, 1977.

55. Pakrashi, A., and Shaha, C., Anti-implantation and anti-oestrogenic activity of a sesquiterpene from the roots of *Aristolochia indica* Linn., *Indian J. Exp. Biol.*, 15, 1197, 1977.

56. Pakrashi, A., and Chakrabarty, B., Antifertility effect of aristolic acid from *Aristolochia indica* Linn. in female albino rabbits, *Experientia*, 34, 1377, 1978.

57. Pakrashi, A., and Chakrabarty, B., Anti-oestrogenic and anti-implantation effect of aristolic acid from *Aristolochia indica* Linn., *Indian J. Exp. Biol.*, 16, 1283, 1978.

58. Pakrashi, S.C., Ghosh-Dastidar, P., Basu, S., and Achari, B., New phenanthrene derivatives from *Aristolochia indica*, *Phytochemistry*, 16, 1103, 1977.

59. Chandhoke, N., Daturalactone (DQ_1) isolated from *Datura quercifolia*: a new interceptive agent, *Indian J. Exp. Biol.*, 16, 419, 1978.

60. Chandhoke, N., Gupta, S., and Dhar, S., Interceptive activity of various species of *Piper*, their natural amides, and semi-synthetic analogs, *Indian J. Pharm. Sci.*, 40, 113, 1978.

61. Chandhoke, N., and Gupta, S., Estrogenic activity of DQ_1 - a steroidal lactone - isolated from *Datura quercifolia*, *Indian J. Exp. Biol.*, 16, 648, 1978.

62. Emmens, C.W., Postcoital contraception, *Brit. Med. Bull.*, 26, 45, 1970.

63. Morris, J.M., and van Wagenen, G., Compounds interfering with ovum implantation and development III: the role of estrogens, *Amer. J. Obstet. Gynecol.*, 96, 804, 1966.

64. Reel, J.R., Humphrey, R.R., Shih, Y.H., Windsor, B.L., Sakowski, R., Creger, P.L., and Edgren, R.A., Competitive progesterone antagonists: receptor binding and biologic activity of testosterone and 19-nortestosterone derivatives, *Fert. Steril.*, 31, 552, 1979.

65. Kholkute, S.D., and Udupa, K.N., Antiestrogenic activity of *Hibiscus rosa-sinensis* Linn. flowers, *Indian J. Exp. Biol.*, 14, 175, 1976.

66. Kholkute, S.D., and Udupa, K.N., Effects of *Hibiscus rosa-sinensis* on pregnancy of rats, *Planta Med.*, 29, 321, 1976.

67. Kholkute, S.D., Mudgal, V., and Udupa, K.N., Studies on the antifertility potentiality of *Hibiscus rosa-sinensis*, *Planta Med.*, 31, 35, 1977.

68. Kholkute, S.D., Mudgal, V., and Deshpande, P.J., Screening of indigenous medicinal plants for antifertility potentiality, *Planta Med.*, 29, 151, 1976.

69. Batta, S.K., and Santhakumari, G., The antifertility effect of *Ocimum sanctum* and *Hibiscus rosa-sinensis*, *Indian J. Med. Res.*, 59, 777, 1971.

70. Kholkute, S.D., Srivastava, D.N., Chatterjee, S., and Udupa, K.N., Effects of some compounds isolated from *Hibiscus rosa-sinensis* flowers on pregnancy in rats, *J. Res. Indian Med. Yoga Homoeopathy*, 11, 106, 1976.

71. Razdan, M.K., Kapila, K., and Bhide, N.K., Antifertility effect and some pharmacological actions of *Butea frondosa* seed extracts, *Indian J.*

Physiol. Pharmacol., 13, 239, 1969.

72. Tewari, P.V., Mapa, H.C., and Chaturvedi, C., Experimental study on estrogenic activity of certain indigenous drugs, *J. Res. Indian Med. Yoga Homoeopathy*, 11, 7, 1976.

73. Kapila, K., Bhide, N.K., and Razdan, M.K., The antifertility effect of *Butea frondosa* petals (alcoholic extract and its crystalline fraction), *J. Indian Med. Ass.*, 55, 60, 1970.

74. Laumas, K.R., and Uniyal, J.P., A preliminary report on the antiestrogenic activity of the petals of *Butea frondosa* flowers, *Indian J. Exp. Biol.*, 4, 246, 1966.

75. Garg, S.K., Mathur, V.S., and Chaudhury, R.R., Screening of Indian plants for antifertility activity, *Indian J. Exp. Biol.*, 16, 1077, 1978.

76. Prakash, A.O., and Mathur, R., Screening of Indian plants for antifertility activity, *Indian J. Exp. Biol.*, 14, 623, 1976.

77. Arora, R.B., Ghatak, N., and Gupta, S.P., Antifertility activity of *Embelia ribes*, *J. Res. Indian Med.*, 6, 107, 1971.

78. Kholkute, S.D., Kekare, M.B., Jathar, V.S., and Munshi, S.R., Antifertility effects of *Embelia ribes* Burm., *Indian J. Exp. Biol.*, 16, 1035, 1978.

79. Rathinam, K., Santhakumari, G., and Ramiah, N., Studies on the antifertility activity of embelin, *J. Res. Indian Med. Yoga Homoeopathy*, 11, 84, 1976.

80. Radhakrishnan, N., and Alam, M., Antifertility activity of embelin in albino rats, *Indian J. Exp. Biol.*, 13, 70, 1975.

81. Radhakrishnan, N., and Alam, M.M., Antiestrogenic action of embelin, *J. Res. Indian Med. Yoga Homoeopathy*, 11, 115, 1976.

82. Prakash, A.O., Effect of *Embelia ribes* on uterine weight of normal and ovariectomized rats, *Planta Med.*, 35, 370, 1979.

83. Prakash, A.O., and Mathur, R., Studies on oestrous cycle of albino rats: response to *Embelia ribes* extracts, *Planta Med.*, 36, 134, 1979.

84. Kholkute, S.D., Kekare, M.B., and Munshi, S.R., Antifertility effects of the fruits of *Piper longum* in female rats, *Indian J. Exp. Biol.*, 17, 289, 1979.

85. Matsui, A. de S., Hoskin, S., Kashiwagi, M., Aguda, B.W., Zegart, B.E., Norton, I.R., and Cutting, W.C., A survey of natural products from Hawaii and other areas of the Pacific for an antifertility effect in mice, *Int. Z. Klin. Pharmakol. Ther. Toxikol.*, 5, 65, 1971.

86. Gujral, M.L., Varma, D.R., and Sareen, K.N., Oral contraceptives, part I: preliminary observations on the antifertility effect of some indigenous drugs, *Indian J. Med. Res.*, 48, 46, 1960.

87. Gujral, M.L., Varma, D.R., Sareen, K.N., and Roy, A.K., Oral contraceptives, part II: antifertility effect of *Mallotus philippinensis* Mueller-Argoviensis, *Indian J. Med. Res.*, 48, 52, 1960.

88. Khanna, U., and Chaudhury, R.R., Antifertility screening of plants, part I: investigations on *Butea monosperma* (Lam.) Kuntze., *Indian J. Med. Res.*, 56, 1575, 1968.

89. Khanna, U., Garg, S.K., Vohora, S.B., Walia, H.B., and Chaudhury, R.R., Antifertility screening of plants, part II: effect of six indigenous plants on early pregnancy in albino rats, *Indian J. Med. Res.*, 57, 237, 1969.

90. Vohora, S.B., Garg, S.K., and Chaudhury, R.R., Antifertility screening of plants, part III: effect of six indigenous plants on early pregnancy in albino rats, *Indian J. Med. Res.*, 57, 893, 1969.

91. Garg, S.K., Vohora, S.B., and Chaudhury, R.R., Antifertility screening of plants, part IV: investigations on *Butea monosperma* (Lam.) Kuntze.,

Indian J. Med. Res., 57, 1946, 1969.

92. Saksena, S.K., Garg, S.K., and Chaudhury, R.R., Antifertility screening of plants, part V: effect of six indigenous plants on early pregnancy in albino rats, *Indian J. Med. Res.*, 58, 253, 1970.

93. Garg, S.K., Saksena, S.K., and Chaudhury, R.R., Antifertility screening of plants, part VI: effect of five indigenous plants on early pregnancy in albino rats, *Indian J. Med. Res.*, 58, 1285, 1970.

94. Garg, S.K., and Garg, G.P., Antifertility screening of plants, part VII: effect of five indigenous plants on early pregnancy in albino rats, *Indian J. Med. Res.*, 59, 302, 1971.

95. Garg, S.K., Antifertility screening of plants, part VIII: investigation on *Taxus baccata* Linn. leaves, *Indian J. Med. Res.*, 60, 159, 1972.

96. Garg, S.K., and Mathur, V.S., Effect of chromatographic fractions of *Polygonum hydropiper* Linn. (roots) on fertility in female albino rats, *J. Reprod. Fert.*, 29, 421, 1972.

97. Garg, S.K., and Mathur, V.S., Effect of chromatographic fractions of *Daucus carota* Linn. (seeds) on fertility in female albino rats, *J. Reprod. Fert.*, 31, 143, 1972.

98. Bodhankar, S.L., Garg, S.K., and Mathur, V.S., Antifertility screening of plants, part IX: effect of five indigenous plants on early pregnancy in female albino rats, *Indian J. Med. Res.*, 62, 831, 1974.

99. Garg, S.K., Antifertility effect of oil from a few indigenous plants on female albino rats, *Planta Med.*, 26, 391, 1974.

100. Moser, M.B., Seri: from conception through infancy, *The Kiva*, 35, 201, 1970.

101. Powell, J.M., Ethnobotany, in *New Guinea Vegetation*, Paijmans, K., Ed., Elsevier Scientific Publishing Co., Amsterdam, 1976, 147.

102. Arenas, P., and Moreno-Azorero, R., Plants used as means of abortion, contraception, sterilization, and fecundation by Paraguayan indigenous people, *Econ. Bot.*, 31, 302, 1977.

103. Latorre, D.L., and Latorre, F.A., Plants used by the Mexican Kickapoo Indians, *Econ. Bot.*, 31, 340, 1977.

104. Moore, M., *Los Remedios de la Gente*, M. Moore, Publisher, Santa Fe, 1977, 8.

105. Garg, S.K., Antifertility effect of some chromatographic fractions of *Daucus carota*, *Indian J. Pharmacol.*, 7, 40, 1975.

106. Garg, S.K., Antifertility screening of plants - effect of four indigenous plants on early pregnancy in female albino rats, *Indian J. Med. Res.*, 64, 1133, 1976.

107. Garg, S.K., Effect of *Curcuma longa* (rhizomes) on fertility in experimental animals, *Planta Med.*, 26, 225, 1974.

108. Morris, J.M., Postcoital antifertility agents and their teratogenic effect, *Contraception*, 2, 85, 1970.

109. Thiersch, J.B., The control of reproduction in rats with the aid of antimetabolites and early experiences with antimetabolites as abortifacient agents in man, *Acta Endocrinol. Suppl.*, 28, 37, 1956.

110. Morris, J.M., van Wagenen, G., Hurteau, G.D., Johnston, D.W., and Carlsen, R.A., Compounds interfering with ovum implantation and development I: alkaloids and antimetabolites, *Fert. Steril.*, 18, 7, 1967.

111. Wiesner, B.P., and Yudkin, J., Control of fertility by antimitotic agents, *Nature* (London), 176, 249, 1955.

112. Thiersch, J.B., Effect of *N*-desacetylthiocolchicine (TC) and *N*-desacetylmethylcolchicine (MC) on rat fetus and litter *in utero*, *Proc. Soc. Exp. Biol. Med.*, 98, 479, 1958.

113. Thiersch, J.B., Effect of podophyllin (P) and podophyllotoxin (PT) on the rat litter *in utero*, *Proc. Soc. Exp. Biol. Med.*, 113, 124, 1963.

114. Cohlan, S.Q., Dancis, J., and Kitay, D., Vinblastine, *Lancet*, 1, 1390, 1964.

115. Ferm, V.H., Congenital malformations in hamster embryos after treatment with vinblastine and vincristine, *Science*, 141, 426, 1963.

116. Sieber, S.M., Whang-Peng, J., Botkin, C., and Knutsen, T., Teratogenic and cytogenetic effects of some plant-derived antitumor agents (vincristine, colchicine, maytansine, VP-16-213, and VM-26) in mice, *Teratology*, 18, 31, 1978.

117. Schvartzman, J.B., Benitez, Z., and Moreno-Azorero, R., Accion citostatica de una planta medicinal paraguaya con probable efecto abortivo: *Aristolochia triangularis* Cham., *Rev. Soc. Cient. Paraguay*, 15, 27, 1975.

118. Brazeau, P., Oxytocics: oxytocin, prostaglandins, and ergot alkaloids, in *The Pharmacological Basis of Therapeutics*, 5th ed., Goodman, L.S., and Gilman, A., Eds., Macmillan Publishing Co., Inc., New York, 1975, chap. 42.

119. Hillier, K., Uterine contractility, *J. Appl. Med.*, Dec., 1177, 1977.

120. Speroff, L., Glass, R.H., and Kase, N.G., *Clinical Gynecologic Endocrinology and Infertility*, 2nd ed., The Williams & Wilkins Co., Baltimore, 1978, chap. 5.

121. Morton, J.F., Medicinal and other plants used by people on North Caicos (Turks and Caicos Islands, West Indies), *Q. J. Crude Drug Res.*, 15, 1, 1977.

122. Devereux, G., *A Study of Abortion in Primitive Societies*, Revised ed., International Universities Press, Inc., New York, 1976, 414 pp.

123. Benirschke, K., Cytogenetics, in *Reproductive Endocrinology: Physiology, Pathophysiology, and Clinical Management*, Yen, S.S.C., and Jaffe, R.B., Eds., W.B. Saunders Co., Philadelphia, 1978, chap. 9.

124. Gran, L., On the effect of a polypeptide isolated from "Kalata-Kalata" (*Oldenlandia affinis* DC.) on the oestrogen dominated uterus, *Acta Pharmacol. Toxicol.*, 33, 400, 1973.

125. Turner, R.A., *Screening Methods in Pharmacology*, Academic Press, New York, 1965, chap. 9.

126. Tewari, P.V., Sharma, P.V., and Prasad, D.N., Experimental studies on the ecbolic properties of *Gloriosa superba* Linn. (Kalihāri), *J. Res. Indian Med.*, 7, 27, 1972.

127. Bhatia, B.B., and Lal, S., The pharmacological action of *Plumbago zeylanica* and its active principle (plumbagin), *Indian J. Med. Res.*, 20, 777, 1933.

128. Ko, K., On the pharmacological action of plumbagin, *Jap. J. Med. Sci. Pharmacol.*, 6, 259, 1933.

129. Premakumari, P., Rathinam, K., and Santhakumari, G., Antifertility activity of plumbagin, *Indian J. Med. Res.*, 65, 829, 1977.

130. Asdell, S.A., *Patterns of Mammalian Reproduction*, 2nd ed., Cornell University Press, Ithaca, 1964, pp. 274, 311, and 363.

131. Hu, S.Y., A contribution to our knowledge of *Leonurus* L., I-mu-ts'ao, the Chinese motherwort, *J. Chin. Univ. Hong Kong*, 2, 365, 1974.

132. Kong, Y.C., and Yeung, H.W., Effect of the Chinese motherwort (*Leonurus artemisia*) on mammalian reproductive function, *Chung Chi J.*, 13, 25, 1974.

133. Kong, Y.C., Hu, S.Y., Hwang, J.C., Chan, S.H.H., and Yeung, H.W., Studies on I-mu-ts'ao - an introductory report, *J. Chin. Univ. Hong*

Kong, 2, 345, 1974.

134. Kong, Y.C., Yeung, H.W., Cheung, Y.M., and Hwang, J.C., Isolation of the uterotonic principle from *Leonurus artemisia*, the Chinese motherwort, *Amer. J. Chin. Med.*, 4, 373, 1976.

135. Yeung, H.W., Kong, Y.C., Lay, W.P., and Cheng, K.F., The structure and biological effect of leonurine, *Planta Med.*, 31, 51, 1977.

136. Cheng, K.F., Yip, C.S., Yeung, H.W., and Kong, Y.C., Leonurine, an improved synthesis, *Experientia*, 35, 571, 1979.

137. Gran, L., 5-Hydroxytryptamine (serotonin) isolated from *Oldenlandia affinis*, *Medd. Nor. Farm. Selsk.*, 34, 125, 1972.

138. Gran, L., Oxytocic principles of *Oldenlandia affinis*, *Lloydia*, 36, 174, 1973.

139. Lipton, A., An active glycoside from *Albizia* species and its action on isolated uterus and ileum, *J. Pharm. Pharmacol.*, 15, 816, 1963.

140. Rendle-Short, C.W., Rupture of the gravid uterus in Uganda, *Amer. J. Obstet. Gynecol.*, 79, 1114, 1960.

141. Lipton, A., Physiological activity in extracts of *Albizia* species, *Nature* (London), 184, 822, 1959.

142. Lipton, A., Effects on anaesthetised animals of an oxytocic glycoside extracted from certain species of *Albizia*, *J. Pharm. Pharmacol.*, 16, 369, 1964.

143. Lipton, A., Abortifacient and toxic actions of the glycoside 'albitocin' extracted from some *Albizia* species, *J. Pharm. Pharmacol.*, 19, 792, 1967.

144. Levine, S.D., Adams, R.E., Chen, R., Cotter, M.L., Hirsch, A.F., Kane, V.V., Kanojia, R.M., Shaw, C., Wachter, M.P., Chin, E., Huettemann, R., and Ostrowski, P., Zoapatanol and montanol, novel oxepane diterpenoids,

from the Mexican plant zoapatle (*Montanoa tomentosa*), *J. Amer. Chem. Soc.*, 101, 3404, 1979.

145. Kanojia, R.M., U.S. Patent 4,060,604, 1977.

146. Mateos, J.L., Noriega, L., Huettemann, R.E., and Kanojia, R.M., U.S. Patent 3,996,132, 1976.

147. The Second Laboratory, Shanghai Institute of Experimental Biology, Studies on the mechanisms of abortion induction by trichosanthin, *Sci. Sin.*, 19, 811, 1976.

148. Shanghai Trichosanthin Research Group, 200 Cases of induced abortion by trichosanthin injection, *Chin. Med. J.*, 56, 215, 1976.

149. Wang, Y., Ling, J., and Zhu, L., Preliminary studies on purification and characterization of an abortifacient plant protein, trichosanthin, *Acta Zool. Sin.*, 22, 137, 1976.

150. Hsu, K., Jiang, W., Chen, Y., and Huang, M., Studies on the site of action of induced abortion by trichosanthin, *Acta Zool. Sin.*, 22, 149, 1976.

151. Zhu, Y., and Cai, S., Studies on the relationship between endogenous synthesis of prostaglandins and abortion induction by trichosanthin, *Acta Zool. Sin.*, 22, 180, 1976.

152. Xiong, Y., Zhang, J., Xu, S., Pan, P., and Wang, Y., Preliminary study on the relationship between the immunogenic inhibition by phenergan and the termination of pregnancy by trichosanthin, *Acta Zool. Sin.*, 22, 187, 1976.

153. Su, H.T., Wei, H., Wu, B.Y., and Lu, Y.Q., Effect of radix *Trichosanthis* injection on uterus contraction of early pregnant rabbits, *Acta Physiol. Sin.*, 31, 21, 1979.

154. Wang, Y., Ju, R., Huang, J., and Hsu, K., Investigations on the

injurious effects of the abortifacient trichosanthin to monkey placental villi, *Acta Zool. Sin.*, 22, 156, 1976.

155. Wang, Y.T., Hsu, K.C., and Chiang, W.S., The ultrastructural observations on the injurious effects of the abortifacient trichosanthin on monkey trophoblast, *Acta Biol. Exp. Sin.*, 11, 263, 1978.

156. Cao, M., Liang, S., Luo, R., He, Q., Shi, A., and Jin, Y., The distribution and mode of excretion of the ^{131}I-labeled crude extract of radix *Trichosanthis* in pregnant women, *Acta Zool. Sin.*, 22, 144, 1976.

157. Tso, J., Liu, S., and Liu, L., Serum HCG levels of women during and after abortion induced by trichosanthin, *Acta Zool. Sin.*, 22, 166, 1976.

158. Xiong, Y., Pan, P., Xu, S., Zhang, J., Wang, Y., Zuo, J., and Gu, Z., Study on the effects of trichosanthin on human trophoblast cells *in vitro*, *Acta Zool. Sin.*, 22, 172, 1976.

159. Jiang, T., Gao, K., Zhou, G., Zhu, Y., and Cai, H., Changes in urinary pregnanediol and estriol excretions during second trimester abortion induced by trichosanthin - a protein extracted from radix trichosanthei, *Acta Zool. Sin.*, 23, 243, 1977.

160. Tso, J.K., Wang, Y.P., and Wang, M.P., Analysis of effects of trichosanthin on the function of syncytiotrophoblasts, *Acta Biol. Exp. Sin.*, 11, 277, 1978.

161. Coleman, S., and Piotrow, P.T., Spermicides - simplicity and safety are major assets, *Pop. Rep.*, Series H, 77, 1979.

162. Setty, B.S., Kamboj, V.P., and Khanna, N.M., Screening of Indian plants for biological activity, part VII: spermicidal activity of Indian plants, *Indian J. Exp. Biol.*, 15, 231, 1977.

163. Setty, B.S., Kamboj, V.P., Garg, H.S., and Khanna, N.M., Spermicidal potential of saponins isolated from Indian medicinal plants, *Contra-*

ception, 14, 571, 1976.

164. Jain, G.K., Sarin, J.P.S., and Khanna, N.M., Constitution of scheffleroside - a spermicidal saponin from *Schefflera capitata*, *Indian J. Chem.*, 15B, 1139, 1977.

165. Stolzenberg, S.J., and Parkhurst, R.M., Spermicidal actions of extracts and compounds from *Phytolacca dodecandra*, *Contraception*, 10, 135, 1974.

166. Varshney, I.P., and Khanna, N., Partial structure of a new saponin samanin-D from the flowers of *Pithecellobium saman* Benth., *Indian J. Pharm. Sci.*, 40, 60, 1978.

167. Varshney, I.P., Vyas, P., Srivastava, H.C., and Singh, P.P., Study of *Albizia lebbek* Benth. wood saponin, lebbekanin-E, *Nat. Acad. Sci. Lett. (India)*, 2, 135, 1979; through *Chem. Abstr.*, 91, 120369c, 1979.

168. Shaaban, A.H., and Ahmed, Z.F., A new spermicidal principle from *Phytolacca americana* Linn., *Egypt. Soc. Gyn. Obstet.*, 9, 27, 1959.

169. Ericsson, R.J., Male antifertility compounds: U-5897 as a rat chemosterilant, *J. Reprod. Fert.*, 22, 213, 1970.

170. Jackson, H., Chemical interference with spermatogenesis and fertility, in *Advances in Reproductive Physiology*, Vol. 4, McLaren, A., Ed., Logos Press, London, 1969, chap. 2.

171. Vilar, O., Effect of cytostatic drugs on human testicular function, in *Male Fertility and Sterility*, Proc. Serono Symp. Vol. 5, Mancini, R.E., and Martini, L., Eds., Academic Press, London, 1974, 423.

172. Merlin, H.E., Azoospermia caused by colchicine - a case report, *Fert. Steril.*, 23, 180, 1972.

173. Sieber, S.M., and Adamson, R.H., Toxicity of antineoplastic agents in man: chromosomal aberrations, antifertility effects, congenital malformations, and carcinogenic potential, in *Advances in Cancer Research*,

Vol. 22, Klein, G., and Weinhouse, S., Eds., Academic Press, Inc., New York, 1975, 57.

174. Joshi, M.S., and Ambaye, R.Y., Effect of alkaloids from *Vinca rosea* L. on spermatogenesis in male rats, *Indian J. Exp. Biol.*, 6, 256, 1968.

175. Zuckerberg, C., and Solari, A.J., Centriolar changes induced by vinblastine sulphate in the seminiferous epithelium of the mouse, *Exp. Cell Res.*, 76, 470, 1973.

176. Bustos-Obregon, E., and Feito, R., The effect of vinblastine sulfate on rat spermatogenesis, *Arch. Biol. (Bruxelles)*, 85, 353, 1974.

177. Parvinen, L.M., Söderström, K.O., and Parvinen, M., Early effects of vinblastine and vincristine on the rat spermatogenesis: analyses by a new transillumination-phase contrast microscopic method, *Exp. Pathol.*, 15, 85, 1978.

178. Lee, I.P., and Dixon, R.L., Effects of vincristine on spermatogenesis studied by velocity sedimentation cell separation technique and serial mating, *J. Pharmacol. Exp. Ther.*, 181, 192, 1972.

179. Pakrashi, A., and Pakrasi, P.L., Antispermatogenic effect of the extract of *Aristolochia indica* Linn. on male mice, *Indian J. Exp. Biol.*, 15, 256, 1977.

180. Kholkute, S.D., Effect of *Hibiscus rosa-sinensis* on spermatogenesis and accessory reproductive organs in rats, *Planta Med.*, 31, 127, 1977.

181. Dixit, V.P., Effects of *Malvaviscus conzattii* Greenm. flower extract on testicular function of the house rat *Rattus rattus* Rufescens and the gerbil *Meriones hurrianae* Jerdon: a biochemical study, *Indian J. Exp. Biol.*, 15, 506, 1977.

182. Dixit, V.P., and Bhargava, S.K., Effects of *Malvaviscus conzattii* Greenm. flower extract on the male reproductive organs of bat (*Rhinopoma*

kinneari Wroughton): a confirmation, *Proc. Indian Nat. Sci. Acad.*, B44, 1, 1978.

183. Dixit, V.P., Khanna, P., and Bhargava, S.K., Effects of *Momordica charantia* L. fruit extract on the testicular function of dog, *Planta Med.*, 34, 280, 1978.

184. MacLeod, J., and Gold, R.Z., The male factor in fertility and infertility VI: semen quality and certain other factors in relation to ease of conception, *Fert. Steril.*, 4, 10, 1953.

185. Glass, R.H., Infertility, in *Reproductive Endocrinology: Physiology, Pathophysiology, and Clinical Management*, Yen, S.S.C., and Jaffe, R.B., Eds., W.B. Saunders Co., Philadelphia, 1978, chap. 19.

186. Barfield, A., Melo, J., Coutinho, E., Alvarez-Sanchez, F., Faundes, A., Brache, V., Leon, P., Frick, J., Bartsch, G., Weiske, W.H., Brenner, P., Mishell Jr., D., Bernstein, G., and Ortiz, A., Pregnancies associated with sperm concentrations below 10 million/ml in clinical studies of a potential male contraceptive method, monthly depot medroxyprogesterone acetate and testosterone esters, *Contraception*, 20, 121, 1979.

187. Sanyal, S.N., Oral contraceptive *m*-xylohydroquinone: biological studies on males, *J. Med. Int. Med. Abstr.*, 22, 19, 1958.

188. Sanyal, S.N., and Rana, M., Oral contraceptive - clinical trial with human males with *m*-xylohydroquinone: a preliminary note, *J. Med. Int. Med. Abstr.*, 23, 33, 1959.

189. Sanyal, S.N., Sterility effect of *Pisum sativum* Linn., chemical study IV, *Calcutta Med. J.*, 49, 343, 1952.

190. de Peyster, A., and Wang, Y.Y., Gossypol - proposed contraceptive for men passes the Ames test, *N. Engl. J. Med.*, 301, 275, 1979.

191. National Coordinating Group on Male Antifertility Agents, Gossypol - a

new antifertility agent for males, *Chin. Med. J.*, NS4, 417, 1978.

192. Link, R.P., Toxic plants, rodenticides, herbicides, and yellow fat disease, in *Diseases of Swine*, 4th ed., Dunne, H.W., and Lemon, A.D., Eds., Iowa State University Press, Ames, 1975, chap. 43.

193. Flück, H., The influence of the soil on the content of active principles in medicinal plants, *J. Pharm. Pharmacol.*, 6, 153, 1954.

194. Woodward, E.F., and Smith, E., The acquisition and variability of investigational plant material, *Lloydia*, 25, 281, 1962.

195. Ruhr, L.P., Osweiler, G.D., and Foley, C.W., The effect of zearalenone on fertility in the boar, *Amer. Ass. Vet. Lab. Diag.*, 21, 127, 1978.

196. Jackson, R.A., Fenton, S.W., Mirocha, C.J., and Davis, G., Characterization of two isomers of 8'-hydroxyzearalenone and other derivatives of zearalenone, *J. Agr. Food Chem.*, 22, 1015, 1974.

197. Chow, F.H.C., Hanson, K.J., Hamar, D.W., and Udall, R.H., Reproductive failure of mice caused by pine needle ingestion, *J. Reprod. Fert.*, 30, 169, 1972.

198. Chow, F.C., Hamar, D.W., and Udall, R.H., Mycotoxic effect on fetal development: pine needle abortion in mice, *J. Reprod. Fert.*, 40, 203, 1974.

199. Stevenson, A.H., James, L.F., and Call, J.W., Pine needle (*Pinus ponderosa*) induced abortion in range cattle, *Cornell Vet.*, 62, 519, 1972.

200. Bremner, W.J., and Paulsen, C.A., Colchicine and testicular function in man, *N. Engl. J. Med.*, 294, 1384, 1976.

201. Saba, N., Drane, H.M., Hebert, C.N., and Holdsworth, R.J., Seasonal variation in oestrogenic activity, coumestrol, and formononetin content of white clover, *J. Agr. Sci.*, 83, 505, 1974.

202. Bingel, A.S., and Farnsworth, N.R., The "ideal species" for antifer-

tility screening of plants, presented at WHO Task Force Meeting, Mexico City, January 30 to February 1, 1976, 1.

203. Price, J.R., Antifertility agents of plant origin, in *Biological Council Symposium on Agents Affecting Fertility*, Austin, C.R., and Perry, J.S., Eds., J. & A. Churchill Ltd., London, 1965, 3.

204. Pakrashi, A., Basak, B., and Mookerji, N., Search for antifertility agents from indigenous medicinal plants, *Indian J. Med. Res.*, 63, 378, 1975.

205. Institute for Research in Reproduction, Indigenous plant products and Ayurvedic preparations, Report of Work for the Year, Indian Council of Medical Research, Parel, Bombay, 1976, 27.

206. Guttmacher, A.F., *Pregnancy, Birth, and Family Planning*, The New American Library, Inc., New York, 1973, chap. 4.

4. LUTEINIZING HORMONE RELEASING HORMONE AND ANALOGUES: CONCEPTIVE AND CONTRACEPTIVE POTENTIAL

A. Corbin & F.J. Bex

I. Introduction...228

II. Conceptive Aspects...229

A. Treatment of Female Infertility with LHRH and LHRH Agonists 229

B. Treatment of Male Infertility with LHRH and LHRH Agonists 233

C. Future Prospectives 236

III. Contraceptive Aspects...236

A. LHRH Antagonists 236

B. LHRH and LHRH Agonists 246

1. Antifertility potential in the female 246: *a) Effects on female reproductive function 247; b) Mechanism of anti-reproductive effects in the female 252; c) Reversibility of antifertility effects in the female 257; d) Studies in women and future prospectives 258.*

2. Antifertility potential in the male 262: *a) Effects on male reproductive function 262; b) Mechanism of anti-reproductive effects in the male 265; c) Reversibility of antifertility effects in the male 267; d) Future prospectives for LHRH agonists as male contraceptives 269.*

3. Safety studies: secondary pharmacology and preliminary toxicologic evaluation 270.

IV. Conclusions...273

References...277

I. INTRODUCTION

The isolation and identification of luteinizing hormone releasing hormone (LHRH) had immediate and far reaching implications concerning the diagnosis and treatment of infertility. The availability of synthetic LHRH that was identical in physical, chemical and biological properties to the natural peptide has allowed, over the past nine years, the extensive evaluation of these potential applications. However, in terms of the utility that was originally conceived, progress has proceeded more slowly and success has been less complete than initially anticipated. In this regard, LHRH has been found to be a useful diagnostic adjunct to existing methods but not as a primary means of differentiating hypothalamic and hypophysial dysfunction. Moreover, therapeutic use of LHRH in theoretically appropriate situations, such as in treatment of delayed puberty, oligospermia and hypothalamic anovulation, generally has produced discouraging results. The identification by pharmacokinetic studies of the short half-life (≈ 4 min) of LHRH in humans suggested that the problems that were being encountered may be related to inadequate dosages, length of exposure and bioavailability. However, more involved LHRH treatment regimens employing frequent administration or continuous infusion, quite often in conjunction with established therapies, or use of various highly potent and long-acting agonistic derivatives of the parent compound, have done little to improve the success rate of this pro-fertility approach. In fact, it has become apparent that LHRH and its agonists possess a pharmacologic profile that, in marked contrast to initial concepts, is anti-reproductive in nature. Characterization of this paradoxical anti-reproductive property has included, in laboratory studies, the ability of these LH-releasing agents to induce luteolysis and terminate pregnancy, reduce fecundity, retard puberty, and to inhibit spermatogenesis and, in clinical studies, inhibition of ovulation and disruption of luteal function. Furthermore, evaluation of a wide variety of LHRH derivatives has revealed a direct correlation between agonist (LH release) and anti-reproductive potencies. This association, aside from explaining the limited success of their pro-fertility application, has generated considerable interest in the agonists as a new class of potential contraceptive agents. It is ironic, not only that substances originally thought of as promoting fertility are now being developed as fertility regulators, but that progress towards this latter end has far surpassed that of the LHRH antagonists, which represented the initial LHRH subclass to receive attention for this purpose. In this regard, the most potent antagonists that have emerged from this ongoing synthetic effort require much more material (15-30 times) to inhibit spontaneous ovulation in rodents than is required for the agonists to exert their luteolytic and pregnancy-terminating effects. Additionally, the antagonists, unlike the agonists, have received little clinical attention and it is unclear whether they will effectively block ovulation without the high doses and restrictive dosing regimens presently necessary for this purpose in laboratory studies.

This report will outline certain of the numerous laboratory and clinical studies undertaken in an effort to develop LHRH and its derivatives as a potential treatment for infertility; and the elucidation of the complex, if not, paradoxical qualities of the LH-releasing peptides and the rapid reproductive pharmacologic evolution of the agonist, in contrast to the antagonist, approach to contraception.

II. CONCEPTIVE ASPECTS

A. Treatment of Female Infertility with LHRH and LHRH Agonists

Within a remarkably short interval following the isolation, purification and identification of LHRH from porcine hypothalami,[1-4] and the demonstration of its LH- and its FSH-releasing activity in man,[5,6] the natural hormone was reported to have been successfully used to induce ovulation (further substantiated by a normal and uneventful pregnancy) in a woman with secondary amenorrhea.[7] Although representing a single case involving a patient who was clomiphene-positive and had received prior pergonal® priming, this report, in view of its significant therapeutic implications, was greeted with understandable enthusiasm and optimism. The availability of synthetic LHRH with equivalent biological activity enabled extensive evaluation of the potential utility of this substance in treating a variety of anovulatory conditions.[8,9] Due to the immature follicular status of patients presenting with amenorrhea, it was not entirely unexpected, in the absence of steps to ensure follicular development, that LHRH given as solitary, isolated treatment (single injection; multiple injections or infusion over a limited interval) proved relatively ineffective in inducing ovulation.[10-16] In an effort to provide follicles of sufficient maturity to respond to the exogenous LHRH ovulatory stimulus, subsequent studies utilized established clomiphene or HMG (pergonal®) stimulatory treatment regimens or attempted to induce follicular growth with chronic LHRH treatment, alone or in combination with clomiphene. LHRH, by itself, produced limited success as a maturational stimulus.[17-21] Also, there was no clear association between evidence of follicular stimulation (i.e. increased urinary estrogen levels) and ovulatory response[17] and the resulting ovulatory rate was disappointingly low.[15,19,20] A greater frequency of ovulation in response to an LHRH stimulus was achieved when follicular maturation was induced by clomiphene or HMG, with or without concomitant LHRH.[12,15,19,22,23] Nevertheless, the incidence of successful ovulation represented little, if any, improvement over that expected from existing procedures (clomiphene/HMG/HCG) in a similar patient population. In fact, it was suggested that many of these successes may have occurred spontaneously or as a result of the adjunct therapies and not LHRH.[9] However, there was continued interest in the development of an LHRH-based therapy since this compound had not been found to produce hyperstimulation even in the presence of exaggerated follicular growth and might, therefore, alleviate the multiple ovulation complications frequently associated with traditional hCG ovulatory therapies.[7,20,21] Moreover, treatment with LHRH was observed, in certain cases, to restore clomiphene responsiveness.[24]

Ongoing synthetic efforts identified a number of LHRH derivatives with much greater potency and duration of activity than the parent compound.[25-27] It was suggested that these analogs might produce the prolonged elevation of LH and more importantly, FSH levels, considered necessary for complete follicular development and, administered acutely, might stimulate a gonadotropin pattern which more closely resembled that necessary for successful ovulation. Chronic use of one such analog, D-Ala^{6}-Des-Gly^{10}-Pro^{9}-NHEt-LHRH, reestablished menstrual cyclicity in 3 of the 7 women treated for secondary amenorrhea but there were no positive signs of ovulation.[28] Similarly, it was reported that in spite of the occurrence of menstruation (in certain individuals during post-treatment cycles), in 9 of 13 patients receiving D-Ala^{6}-LHRH propylamide, none of the treatment cycles appeared to be ovulatory.[29] While ovulation was detected in only 4 out of 20 amenorrheic women administered various regimens of either of two equipotent LHRH agonistic analogs (D-Ala^{6}-Des-Gly^{10}-NHEt-LHRH; D-Leu^{6}-Des-Gly^{10}-NHEt-LHRH), breakthrough bleeding or withdrawal bleeding occurred in a majority of the patients.[9] Treatment of amenorrheic women with D-Ser(TBu)^{6}-Des-Gly^{10}-Pro^{9}-NHEt-LHRH produced either transient estrogen[30] or variable[31] changes in estradiol concentrations and occasional breakthrough or withdrawal bleeding, but no signs of spontaneous menstruation, follicular maturation or ovulation were observed. More encouraging results were reported in two studies employing D-Trp^6-LHRH where ovulation was induced in a total of 7 out of 14 previously anovulatory women; in 5 of these subjects pregnancy was achieved.[32,33]

Quite possibly, the heterogeneous etiology of the anovulatory states in which LHRH, and later, the agonistic analogs have been employed, has obscured their utility as follicular maturational and ovulation-inducing agents. However, it is clear that their successful therapeutic application is far more circumscribed than initially foreseen and further patient classification will be necessary before appropriate indications and associated treatment regimens can be recommended. Moreover, the use of LHRH to diagnose those conditions which would be benefitted most by LHRH treatment has proven less successful than anticipated. Instead of representing a principle means of differentiating hypothalamic from pituitary disease, it appears that its major utility is as an adjunct to established diagnostic procedures.[8,34-38]

Development of successful pro-fertility regimens utilizing the potent and long-acting LHRH agonists may be further complicated by the possibility of reduced pituitary sensitivity (or exhaustion) when these compounds are chronically administered.[31,39] However, it has become increasingly apparent that the major obstacle to therapeutic use may be the paradoxical luteolytic activity of the LH releasing class of peptides first identified in laboratory studies,[40] verified clinically,[41-45] and presently forming the basis for the development of a non-steroidal contraceptive approach. In this regard, review of the various studies, in which LHRH or its agonists were used in treating amenorrheic patients, reveals that in those cases where ovulation was induced the resulting pregnancy rate was exceedingly poor.[8.21,46] In fact, the observation of luteal phase deficiencies following LHRH-stimulated ovulation[19,21,47] has led to the suggestion that progesterone or hCG supplementation may be required for successful therapy.[19,34] Similarly, a large discrepancy between ovulation and pregnancy rates was observed when LHRH was used in synchronizing ovulation with insemination therapy.[48]

Thus, the persistent problem of achieving sufficient follicular maturation, which was not overcome, as expected, by the use of "super agonist" LHRH analogs, coupled with the paradoxical luteolytic activity of these compounds seriously compromises their potential as a pro-fertility therapy for anovulation and other cycle disturbances.

B. Treatment of Male Infertility with LHRH and LHRH Agonists

Attempts to utilize LHRH and its agonists to treat various hypogonadal states in the male were based on a rationale similar to that in the female. However, as in the female, there have been conflicting reports regarding the success of this therapy and few, if any, firm recommendations either defining the conditions most likely to be benefitted by the LH-releasing peptides or the nature of the treatment regimens that would be most appropriate. Moreover, the limitations of these compounds that were identified in the female, such as pituitary desensitization and anti-gonadal activity, have been found to apply in the male, as well. In fact, these effects may be a greater liability to successful male therapy since the length of exposure that would be required for support during a spermatogenic cycle far exceeds that necessary for follicular maturation and ovulation. However, a majority of the studies involving LHRH or its agonistic analog treatment of idiopathic oligospermic conditions utilized massive daily dosages of compound administered for prolonged intervals generally in excess of a spermatogenic cycle. The initial report of LHRH use in male infertility which employed a total of 1 mg administered daily for 6 months indicated increased but still subnormal sperm counts in the azoospermic recipients and a significant but transient, increase in sperm count in the oligospermic patients despite continued treatment.[49] Administration of a total of 1.5 mg daily for up to a year in a heterogeneous group of infertile patients demonstrated a rapid restoration of potency and, despite a slight increase in total androgens, which did not achieve the normal range, the appearance of spermatogenesis in those subjects treated for more than 4 months.[50] Lower dosages of LHRH (500 μg/day) given for up to 22 weeks increased sperm count in 2 of 4 normogonadotropic oligospermic men in the absence of a consistent change in serum testosterone.[51] It was particularly interesting, in view of confirmation provided by later studies, that all patients reported an increase in libido. By dividing normogonadotropic infertile patients into 2 subgroups on the basis of the extent of their sperm maturational defects, it was found that 4 out of 5 hypospermic men responded to LHRH treatment with increased sperm count, motility, and forward directional movement in contrast to similar improvement in only 1 out of 5 of the more severely impaired subjects.[52] However, long-term administration was required for these positive results and the suggestion was made that at least 90 days of 250 μg LHRH/day would offer the best prospect for therapeutic effectiveness. It was also hypothesized that much more prolonged and greater elevation of LH and FSH induced by LHRH agonists might be effectively used in patients with more severe spermatogenic dysfunction who were resistant to LHRH therapy. In this regard, a study in which the potent analog D-Leu^6-Des-Gly^{10}-Pro^9-NHEt-LHRH was self-administered by patients with isolated gonadotropin deficiency at a dose of 100 μg/day revealed that basal and LHRH-stimulated LH levels were only transiently increased during the first 2 weeks of the 2-month treatment period.[53,54] Concentrations of FSH actually decreased during treatment; no consistent changes were seen in levels of testosterone, and there was no improvement of the hypogonadotropic condition. A similar gonadotropin response was seen during chronic (27-38 weeks) treatment of hypogonadotropic hypogonadal patients with the agonistic analog, D-Ser(TBu)^{6}-Des-Gly^{10}-Pro^{9}-NHEt-LHRH.[55] Initially (within 1 week), gonadotropin levels were increased but declined progressively over the treatment interval, an effect which was attributed to either desensitization of the pituitary or exhaustion of pituitary synthesis and storage capacity. However, an analog of similar potency, D-Trp^{6}-LHRH, administered to hypogonadotropic hypogonadal subjects every 8 hours (10 μg/injection) for more than 3 months, produced a moderate elevation in gonadotropin levels, a slight increase in peripheral testosterone correlating with improvement in Tanner scale ranking, but a modest, if any, stimulation of germinal or Leydig cell growth.[56]

While the agonists may be more likely than LHRH to elicit an LH and FSH response from hypogonadotropic hypogonadal males when administered acutely, it is evident from studies in normal men[57-59] and suggested by studies in infertile men[54,55] that this advantage would be quickly lost during the chronic treatment presumed necessary to support a spermatogenic cycle. The pituitary desensitizing effect of this class of peptides coupled with their increasingly apparent anti-gonadal properties (vide infra) and the, as yet, unclear respective role of the gonadotropins in spermatogenesis necessitates a careful re-evaluation of the agonist approach to treating male infertility.

Additionally, LHRH, as well as an analog, have been used as a substitute for hCG in the treatment of cryptorchidism.[60,61] Recently, pernasal administration of LHRH was shown to successfully induce testicular descent in 16 out of 25 boys within 5 weeks of continuous treatment with 200 μg given 6 times daily.[62] The effectiveness of the treatment was particularly interesting in view of the hormonal correlates during therapy which were reminiscent of pituitary desensitization as evidenced by a transitory increase in LH responsiveness to LHRH stimulation, a significant decrease in FSH responsiveness, and no observable changes in serum testosterone. This success was achieved despite minimal hormonal stimulation; a situation which underscores the complex activity of LHRH and the hormones it regulates as well as the intricacy of their involvement in ensuring normal reproductive function.

C. Future Prospectives

While the use of LHRH as a treatment for infertility has produced conflicting and generally disappointing results, this extensive clinical experience has greatly increased our understanding of the regulation of hypothalamic-pituitary-gonadal function and has revealed the complexity of various dysfunctional states originally thought to be amenable to simple replacement therapy. However, use of highly potent and long-acting LHRH analogs, in view of the recently identified pituitary desensitizing and antifertility properties of this class of peptides has, rather than increasing therapeutic success, quite possibly obscured identification of those situations where a more "physiological" approach would have been more appropriate. In other words, the development of pro-fertility therapy based on the LH-releasing peptides might be more profitably served by attention to other aspects of gonadotropin release such as pulsatile and diurnal patterns as well as the addition of supportive adjunct treatments rather than attaining massive and prolonged gonadotropin release.

III. CONTRACEPTIVE ASPECTS

A. LHRH Antagonists

Initial investigations into the structure-activity relationship of LHRH were concerned primarily with identifying derivatives exhibiting reduced intrinsic activity but retaining the ability to reversibly compete with the parent compound. Theoretically, this antagonistic subclass, by interfering with the activity of the endogenous hormone, would provide a potential means for controlling fertility. While extensive and, as yet, ongoing synthetic programs[26,27] have yielded analogs with progressively increasing inhibitory activity and also have provided much information regarding the primary gonadotropin releasing and binding/conformational portions of the peptide, compounds with potencies sufficient for realistic biological utility, have been identified only quite recently.

The first evidence that dissociation between the binding and secretory processes of LHRH could be achieved was provided by a series of compounds involving deletion of the histidyl residue alone[63] or in combination with modifications which have later been shown to increase resistance of the peptide to inactivation and/or to heighten binding affinity, such as certain D-amino substitutions in the 6 position and deletion of the 10 position glycine coupled with the formation of an N-terminal ethylamide (Fujino modification[64]).[65,66] In fact, the 6 and 10 position modifications have served as the basis for the highly potent and long-acting LHRH agonist class of peptides.

A second generation of antagonists arose from the discovery that a substitution of Phe in the 2 position, by itself, produced a molecule possessing LHRH antagonistic activity.[67] When combined with the metabolically stabilizing D-amino^6 substitution, this inhibitory activity was potentiated.[25,68] Most importantly, these antagonists were the first to be evaluated for their ability to inhibit spontaneous reproductive events (i.e. ovulatory LH surge, ovulation, cyclicity, gestation). This was particularly significant since both *in vitro* and *in vivo* evaluations of antagonistic properties exclusively had employed models which could only indirectly predict antifertility effects. These involved assessing the ability of various potential antagonists to prevent LH release in response to exogenously administered LHRH. The test system

ovariectomized, steroid-blocked rats,[65,66,70-72] immature male rats,[63,66] adult, castrated, estrogen-treated male rats,[63] and intact adult male and female rats.[70] Thus, it was unclear whether the inhibition by the antagonists of a single precisely timed artificial LHRH stimulus, as identified in these models, was predictive of a similar effect on the spontaneous, dynamic release of LHRH/LH and ovulation in the normal cycling animal. In this regard, it has since been demonstrated that not all compounds exhibiting high _in vitro_ antagonist potency have significant anti-ovulatory activity.[73,74] Illustration of this point is provided by the data in Table 1 which reveal that D-Phe^2-D-Ala^6[DesGly^{10}]-Pro^9-NHEt-LHRH and D-Phe^2-D-Ser^6-LHRH are potent inhibitors of LHRH-induced LH release _in vitro_ but possess no anti-ovulatory activity at high dosages. This discrepancy may be partially explained by necessity for quite extensive inhibition of the endogenous ovulatory surge to preclude the minimal LH increase required for ovulation.[75] Moreover, the _in vivo_ effectiveness might be further compromised by the presence of residual agonist (LH-releasing) activity identified for many of these peptides.[76] The compound D-Phe^2-D-Leu^6-LHRH at dosages in hamsters which almost completely suppressed the pre-ovulatory LH and FSH surge was found to have little effect on the ovulatory rate.[77] Although, as seen in Table 1, administration of this D-Phe^2-D-Leu^6-LHRH was able to significantly block ovulation in rats, the massive dosage required not only limited its developmental potential but the increased probability for the expression of its intrinsic LH releasing properties, at these concentrations, seriously questioned whether the necessary maximal inhibition of this reproductive event could be achieved. However, an LHRH derivative, D-Phe^2-D-Ala^6-LHRH, similar in structure and _in vitro_ activity, represented the first novel antagonist to be shown, in the normally cycling,

TABLE 1

Activity of LHRH Antagonists in Cell Culture Compared with *in vivo* Anti-Ovulation and LH Releasing Activity

Structure	Lowest Effective Dose (μg/ml) for Significant *in vitro* LH Inhibition	% Ovulation Inhibition (Rat)	MED 100 Total mg*	*In Vivo* LH Release (Ovax Steroid Blocked Rat)
D-Phe^{2}-D-Arg^{6}-LHRH	0.5	60	6	Slight
[Des-Gly^{10}]-D-Phe^{2}-D-Ala^{6}-Pro^{9}-NHEt-LHRH	1	0	-	NT
D-Phe^{2}-D-Ala^{6}-LHRH	1	100#	3	Slight
D-Phe^{2}-D-Ser^{6}-LHRH	1	0	-	NT
D-Phe^{2}-D-Pgl^{6}-LHRH	1	100	6	NT
D-Phe^{2}-D-Leu^{6}-LHRH	5	80	6	Slight
[Des-His^{2}]-D-Pgl^{6}-LHRH	10	60	6	NT
[Des-His^{2}]-D-Ala^{6}-LHRH	25	0	-	Slight
[Des-His^{2},Gly^{10}]-D-Ala^{6}-Pro^{9}-NHEt-LHRH	100	0+	-	NT
[Des-Trp^{3},Gly^{10}]-D-Ala^{6}-Pro^{9}-NHEt-LHRH	1000	NT	NT	NT

* Highest total dose tested = 6 mg; Rx given as a divided dose every 0.5 h between 1200-1430 h on proestrus; ova search following A.M. (estrus)

NT Not tested

\# Inhibits pre-ovulatory LH surge

\+ Does not inhibit pre-ovulatory LH surge

unanesthetized rat, to significantly depress the pre-ovulatory, proestrous hypophysial LH and FSH surges (Figures 1 and 2), completely inhibit ovulation (Table 1), and prevent pregnancy, pre-coitally, in subsequently inseminated recipients.[68,78,79] Furthermore, suppression of the proestrous LH surge (not FSH) and subsequent ovulation could be obtained by administration of the peptide on the immediately preceding metestrus or diestrus.[80] These extended effects, presumably occurring beyond the compound's active half-life, coupled with the ability of a mating stimulus to potentially override a metestrus- or diestrus-(not proestrus) administered ovulatory block, suggested that there was a neural component to the peptide's activity resembling that observed for the barbiturates. This concept was reinforced by the demonstration that D-Phe^{2}-D-Ala^{6}-LHRH could inhibit the release of endogenous LHRH at the hypothalamic level.[81] Thus, it was apparent that the mechanisms by which the antagonists exert their inhibitory action were more complex than originally anticipated and, most likely because of this, their activities could not easily be predicted by non-physiological (e.g. in vitro) means. Although D-Phe^{2}-D-Ala^{6}-LHRH represented one of the most active of the LHRH derivatives clearly possessing the anti-ovulatory activity crucial to antagonist classification, in laboratory studies the total dosage given over a 2.5-hour period that was required for this effect (12-15 mg/kg) was far greater than that practical for clinical testing, much less clinical utility. Attempts to improve the potency of D-Phe^{2}-D-Ala^{6}-LHRH by either the N-terminal modification or methylating the Ala in the 6 position resulted in a reduction or loss in anti-ovulatory activity.[68,80] In fact, the inability of D-Phe^{2}-D-Ala^{6}-Des-Gly^{10}-Pro^{9}-NHEt-LHRH to block ovulation, despite its superiority over D-Phe^{2}-D-Ala^{6}-LHRH as an in vitro inhibitor of LHRH in a monolayer pituitary culture system, dramatically illustrated the importance of directly assessing the ovulatory endpoint when judging antagonist activity.

Further synthetic efforts revealed that substitutions for the 3 position Trp potentiated the effect of previously established modifications. In this regard, D-Phe^{2}-Phe^{3}-D-Phe^{6}-LHRH was found to be a more potent inhibitor of ovulation than D-Phe^{2}-D-Leu^{6}-LHRH.[82] Although D-Phe^{2}-Phe^{3}-D-Phe^{6}-LHRH offered no advantage in activity over that of D-Phe^{2}-D-Ala^{6}-LHRH, investigation of numerous other compounds with modifications in position 2, 3 and 6 demonstrated that the presence of Pro in position 3 greatly enhanced both *in vitro* and anti-ovulatory potency.[83-86] The triply-substituted analogs, D-Phe^{2}-Pro^{3}-D-Trp^{6}-LHRH and D-Phe^{2}-Pro^{3}-D-Phe^{6}-LHRH were found to inhibit ovulation in the rat at a single subcutaneous injection of 750 µg; representing approximately a 4-fold improvement over that of D-Phe^{2}-D-Ala^{6}-LHRH.[74,85] Constant infusion of 375 µg/day of D-Phe^{2}-Pro^{3}-D-Trp^{6}-LHRH using a minipump completely inhibited ovulation in rats when administered over 4 days.[87]

The observation that the substitution of cyclopentyl carbonyl for pyroGlu^{1} did not affect the *in vitro* antagonist properties of D-Phe^{2}-Pro^{3}-D-Phe^{6}-LHRH suggested this as an additional site that would be amenable to modification.[73] Although this particular tetra-substituted analogue had little anti-ovulatory activity, replacement of pyroGlu^{1} in D-Phe^{2}-D-Trp^{3,6}-LHRH with either Ac-Pro or D-pyroGlu^{1} resulted in the most potent antagonists that had yet been reported and were capable of completely inhibiting ovulation at 200-250 µg/rat.[88,89] Moreover, the prolonged activity of D-pyroGlu^{1}-D-Phe^{2}-D-Trp^{3,6}-LHRH was evidenced by its ability to block ovulation when administered as a single injection either on the morning of proestrus (500 µg/rat) or the afternoon of diestrus (1500 µg/rat).[89] This was also the first antagonist to be reported as capable of inhibiting pregnancy in rats when administered post-coitally.[90]

It has taken nearly eight years of remarkably comprehensive and creative

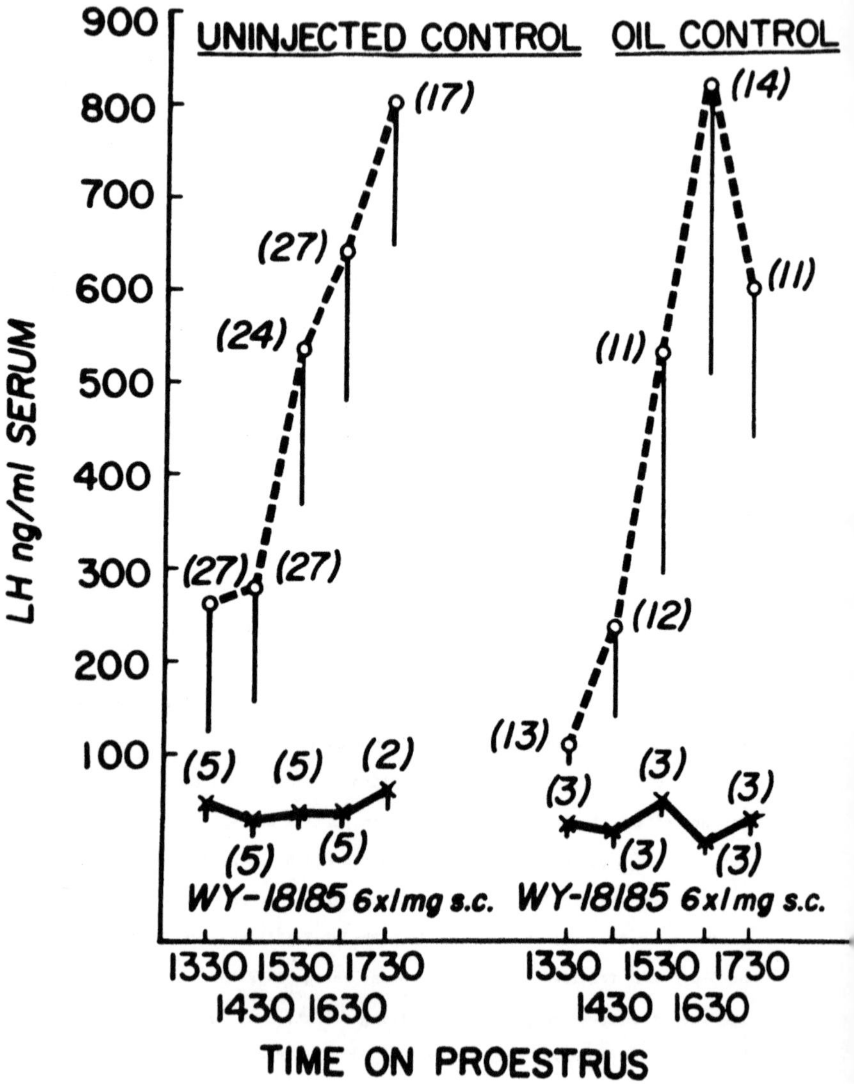

FIG. 1: Effect of the LHRH antagonist, D-Phe^2-D-Ala^6-LHRH (Wy-18,185), on the pre-ovulatory proestrous LH surge: plotted against mean control responses for comparable cycles. ( ) = number of rats/point.

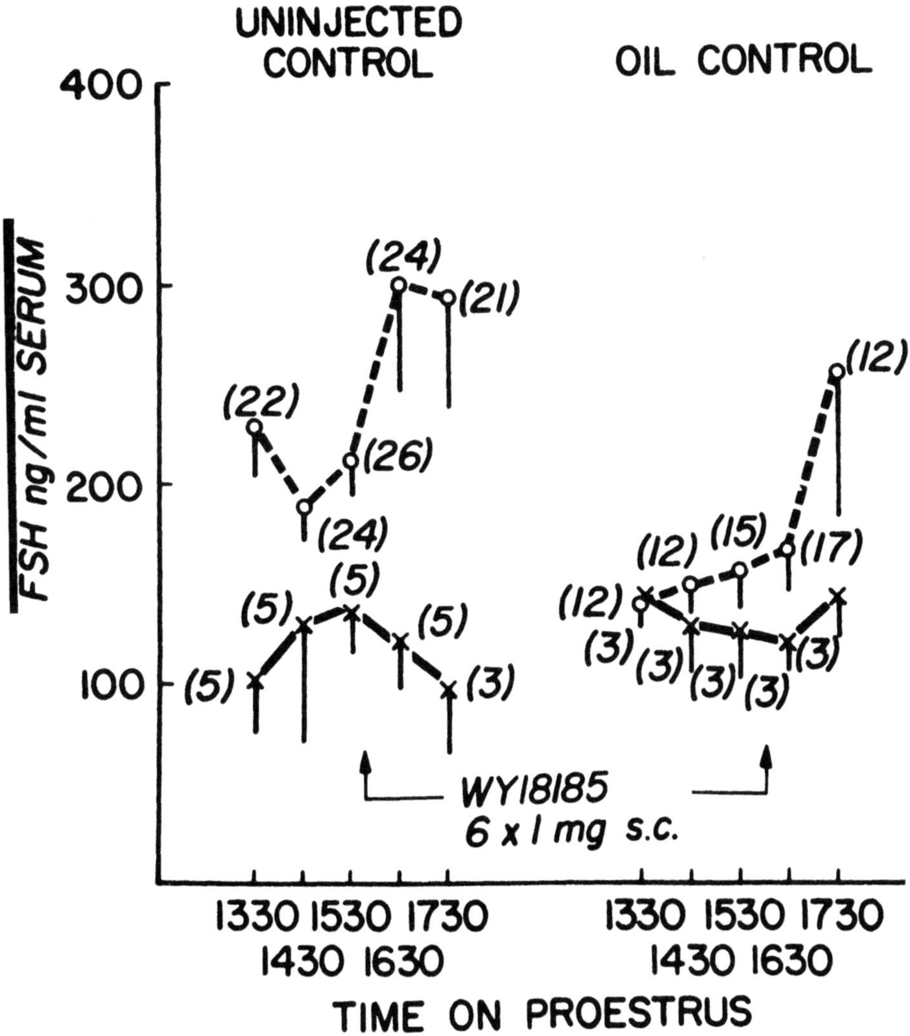

FIG. 2: Effect of the LHRH antagonist, D-Phe^{2}-D-Ala^{6}-LHRH (Wy-18,185), on the pre-ovulatory proestrous FSH surge: plotted against mean control responses for comparable cycles. ( ) = number of rats/point.

synthetic efforts, resulting in literally hundreds of analogs, including such novel antagonists as those containing more than ten residues[91] and those incorporating indomethacin, aspirin or an additional N-terminal pentapeptide sequence (branched pentadecapeptide),[92] to achieve antagonists of the biological potency of D-pyroGlu^{1} and Ac-Pro^{1}-D-Phe^{2}-D-Trp^{3,6}-LHRH.[92a] However, very recently and in rapid succession, a number of additional modifications have been identified which have enabled the production of antagonists with sufficient potencies to consider extensive primate testing. Examples of this latest generation of antagonists and their ovulation-inhibiting activities are shown in Table 2. In view of the increased understanding of the design of antagonists that has been afforded by these developments, coupled with continued extensive synthetic efforts, we anticipate that derivatives will become available in the very near future which will represent at least a 150-fold improvement in ovulation inhibiting potency over the first antagonist shown to affect this endpoint, namely, D-Phe^{2}-D-Ala^{6}-LHRH.

Due to the modest activity and limited quantities of antagonists that had been available, until recently, there has been very little experience with their use in primates. D-Phe^{2}-Phe^{3}-D-Phe^{6}-LHRH and D-Phe^{2}-D-Trp^{3}-D-Phe^{6}-LHRH were found to effectively suppress the release of LH induced by LHRH in the baboon and the chimpanzee, respectively.[93,94] Unfortunately, there has been no test of the effect of these or any other antagonists on spontaneous ovulation or cyclicity in either of these primates. Although D-Phe^{2}-D-Ala^{6}-LHRH was found to be ineffective in altering the length of the menstrual cycle or the quality of cervical mucus when administered prior to expected ovulation in the crab-eating macaque, prior data on the refractoriness of the macaque to LHRH and related agonists suggest that this primate species may be an inappropriate

TABLE 2

LHRH ANTAGONISTS

COMPOUND	OVULATION INHIBITION *MED100, μg/rat, s.c.
(AC-Pro)^{1}-D-Phe^{2}-D-Trp^{3,6}-LHRH	200
(pGlu-Pro)^{1}-D-Phe^{2}-D-Trp^{3,6}-LHRH	200
D-pGlu^{1}-D-Phe^{2}-D-Trp^{3,6}-LHRH	250
D-Phe^{2}-D-Trp^{3}-D-Phe^{6}-LHRH	1500
D-pGlu^{1}-D-Phe^{2}-D-Trp^{3}-D-Phe^{6}-LHRH	350

* APPROXIMATE MINIMUM EFFECTIVE 100% DOSE

model.[95] In men, a massive single intramuscular injection of 90 mg of D-Phe^{2}-D-Trp^{3}-D-Phe^{6}-LHRH effectively attenuated the gonadotropin response to exogenous LHRH[96] but nothing is, as yet, known of the effect of potential antagonists on endogenous reproductive function in humans. While it is hoped that the recent identification of an extremely potent generation of antagonists will allow appropriate clinical evaluation, extensive reproductive ancillary pharmacologic and safety testing must be performed before this class of LHRH derivatives can realistically be considered as the basis for a new method of birth control.

B. LHRH and LHRH Agonists

1. Antifertility Potential in the Female

In addition to their anticipated pro-fertility use, it was proposed that the ovulation inducing properties of LHRH and its agonists might be further exploited to precisely time the fertile period in the normal female and thereby increase the reliability of the rhythm method.

The potent LHRH agonist, D-Ala^{6}-Des-Gly^{10}-Pro^{9}-NHEt-LHRH, was found to advance ovulation and prevent pregnancy in rats.[97,98] The inhibition of pregnancy by the analog was attributed both to disruption of mating behavior and to the occurrence of ovulation at a physiologically inappropriate time. In fact, the possibility that LHRH and agonists may cause release of an immature ovum from a poorly matured follicle was suggested as a potential explanation for the low frequency of pregnancy following their clinical use for ovulation induction.[99] However, more comprehensive evaluation revealed that, apart from the antifertility effects that might be obtained intentionally or unintentionally via their traditionally accepted ovulation-inducing activity, LHRH and its agonists possess very definite anti-reproductive properties. This was first clearly demonstrated by the ability of post-coital administration of LHRH, either pre- or post-implantationally, to disrupt pregnancy in rats.[100] Most importantly, this observation suggested the possibility that this class of peptides might have a much broader application as fertility regulators than that which would be provided by their use in timing ovulation and defining the fertile period.

a) Effects on female reproductive function

In order to investigate the specificity of this seemingly paradoxical contragestational effect of the parent molecule, a large number of LHRH congeners, shown by us or by others[101-102] to have agonistic properties (ovulation induction; LH and/or FSH release in ovariectomized, steroid-blocked rats), were evaluated for their post-coital contraceptive activity.[40,103-107] The potency of these analogs in inducing ovulation (indirect measure of LH-release) was found to be directly correlated with their ability to inhibit pregnancy pre- or post-implantationally (Table 3). The dose-related ability of the two exemplary agonists, D-Trp^{6}-N-MeLeu^{7}-Des-Gly^{10}-Pro^{9}-NHEt-LHRH (Wy-40,972) and D-Ala^{6}-Des-Gly^{10}-Pro^{9}-NHEt-LHRH (Wy-18,481) to inhibit pregnancy in rats, both pre-implantationally (claudogen effect) and post-implantationally (interceptive effect), is depicted in Figures 3 and 4, respectively. The nature of the anti-pregnancy effect produced by these peptides observed on autopsy day 14 following day 1-7 (claudogen) treatment was characterized by a lack of uterine implantation sites or resorption of sites that were present and on autopsy day 18 following day 7-12 (interceptive) treatment by resorbing sites and/or placental scars. Furthermore, this anti-pregnancy activity could be achieved through various modes of administration and, as shown for Wy-40,972 in Table 4, the effectiveness of the route correlated fairly closely with its ovulation-inducing potency. Additionally, the contragestational property of these peptides, as has been quite universally established for their LH-releasing capacity, was found not to be species specific. Either pre- or post-implanta-

TABLE 3

COMPARISON OF THE AGONIST AND POST-COITAL CONTRACEPTIVE PROFILE OF THE [D-Ala^{6}]-LH-RH AND [D-Trp^{6}]-LH-RH SERIES

COMPOUND	AGONIST OVULATION INDUCTION MED_{100^*}, μg/RAT. I.V.	POST-COITAL CONTRACEPTION	
		CLAUDOGEN [MED_{100}, μg/DAY. S.C.]	INTERCEPTIVE
LH-RH	2.0	200-500	500
D-Ala^{6}-LH-RH	1.0	10	100
D-Ala^{6}-Des-Gly^{10}-Pro^{9}-NHEt-LH-RH	1.0	1.0	25-50
D-Ala^{6}-N$^{\alpha}$-Me-Leu^{7}-Des-Gly^{10}-Pro^{9}-NHEt-LH-RH	0.10	1.0	1.0
D-Ala^{6}-N$^{\alpha}$-Me-Leu^{7}-N$^{\alpha}$-Me-Arg^{8}-Des-Gly^{10}-Pro^{9}-NHEt-LH-RH	10	INACTIVE AT 100	INACTIVE AT 100
D-Trp^{6}-LH-RH	0.10	10	1.0-10
D-Trp^{6}-Des-Gly^{10}-Pro^{9}-NHEt-LH-RH	0.10	1.0	10
D-Trp^{6}-N$^{\alpha}$-Me-Leu^{7}-Des-Gly^{10}-Pro^{9}-NHEt-LH-RH	0.10	1.0	~ 1.0
D-Ser(TBU)^{6}-Des-Gly^{10}-Pro^{9}-NHEt-LH-RH (Buserelin)	0.10 - 1.0	10	10

* Approximate minimal effective 100% dose

TABLE 4

OVULATION-INDUCING AND POST-COITAL CONTRACEPTIVE EFFECTS OF WY-40972 VIA VARIOUS ROUTES OF ADMINISTRATION.

ROUTE	OVULATION INDUCING ED^{100}* µg/RAT (SINGLE Rx)	POST-COITAL CONTRACEPTION	
		CLAUDOGEN (D1-7)	INTERCEPTIVE (D7-12)
		ED100, µg/RAT/DAY*	
INTRAVENOUS	0.10	–	–
INTRAMUSCULAR	0.10	10	10
INTRAPERITONEAL	0.10	-	-
SUBCUTANEOUS	>0.10<1.0	1.0	1.0
AEROSOL	10	200	200
TOPICAL	10	-	-
RECTAL	10	-	-
INTRANASAL	10	200	>100<200
ORAL	~10	200	~1000
EAR CANAL	50	-	-
VAGINAL	~50	-	-

* Approximate minimum effective 100% dose.

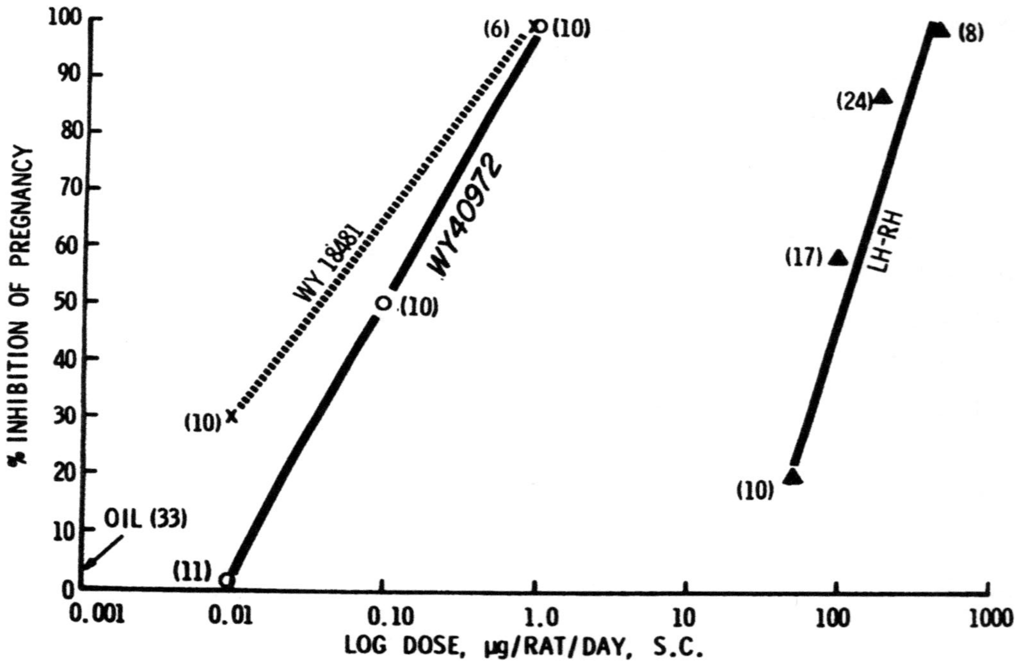

FIG. 3: Post-coital contraceptive effect of LHRH and the LHRH agonists, D-Ala^{6}-Des-Gly^{10}-Pro^{9}-NHEt-LHRH (Wy-18,481) and D-Trp^{7}-N-MeLeu^{7}-Des-Gly^{10}-Pro^{9}-NHEt-LHRH (Wy-40,972), in rats following pre-implantational treatment on days 1-7 of pregnancy. ( ) = number of rats/point.

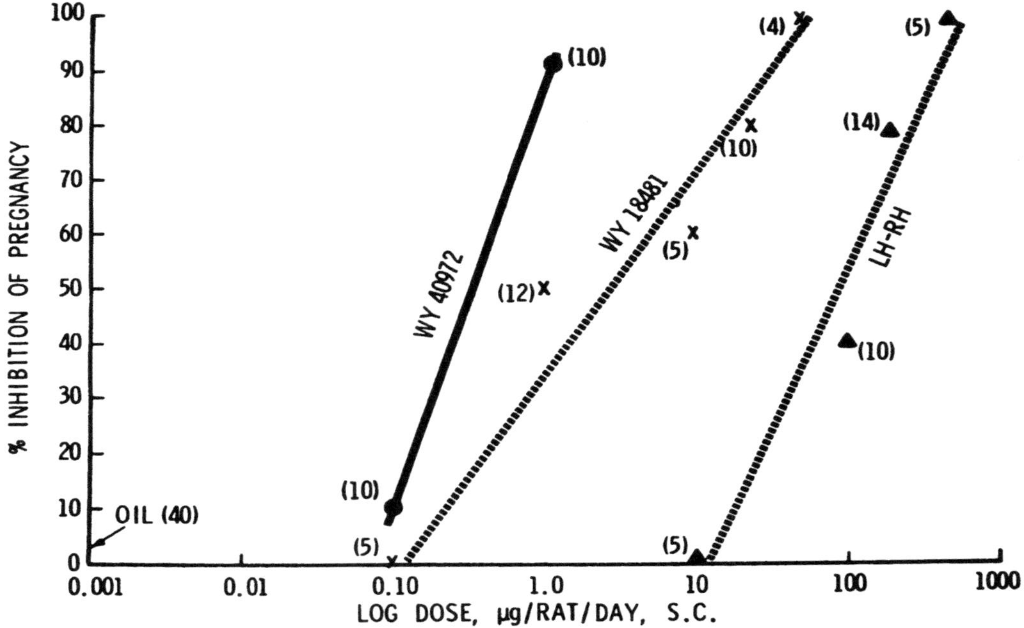

FIG. 4: Post-coital contraceptive effect of LHRH and the LHRH agonists, D-Ala^6-Des-Gly^{10}-Pro^9-NHEt-LHRH (Wy-18,481) and D-Trp^6-N-MeLeu^7-Des-Gly^{10}-Pro^9-NHEt-LHRH (Wy-40,972), in rats following post-implantational treatment on days 7-12 of pregnancy. ( ) = number of rats/point.

tiona.

implantational administration was effective in the hamster.[111]

These paradoxical antifertility effects have been extended and reinforced by the ability of this class of peptides to inhibit other aspects of female reproductive function and development. In pre-coital studies in the rat, acute administration of LHRH was found to disrupt the estrous cycle (delay the onset of estrus and mating) and induce premature ovulation.[97,98,112] Chronic pre-coital administration in the rat, in addition to delaying mating, inhibited pregnancy in a dose-related fashion, and reduced fecundity in those inseminated animals which did deliver. However, the inhibitory effects on pregnancy following pre-coital treatment seem to be due only in part to the observed desynchronization of behavioral and biological events, since ovulation in rats in which the spontaneous ovulatory surge was blocked by pentobarbital, and followed by a normal mating, resulted in only half of the animals becoming pregnant.[106] Thus, these compounds when administered prior to ovulation may directly affect the blastocyst, its transport, or induce luteal incompetency leading to an inappropriate hormonal milieu for implantation and pregnancy in a way similar to their post-coital contragestational action. Evidence for the anti-reproductive effects of the LH-releasing compounds has been extended to pre-pubertal animals as well. Chronic treatment of immature rats with an agonistic analog delayed the time of vaginal opening and retarded the growth of the ovaries, uteri, and anterior pituitary.[106,113-115] It is therefore apparent that the antifertility activity represents the major characteristic and pharmacologic property of this category of peptides in the female, a concept that is supported by data from a variety of experimental models and laboratories employing numerous LHRH congeners.

b) Mechanism of anti-reproductive effects in the female

The possibility that abnormally elevated endogenous LH levels induced by the LH-releasing peptides were responsible for their anti-reproductive effects was first suggested by studies demonstrating the ability of LH to negatively affect ovarian response by reducing its own gonadal receptor levels (down-regulation).[116,117] The likelihood of this mechanism was further reinforced by the direct correlation between capacity to release LH and contragestational activity. Subsequent investigations revealed that either LHRH[118] or its agonists[119,120] did, in fact, produce a dramatic reduction in ovarian, and specifically luteal, LH receptor populations. During pre-implantational treatment, the immediate (within 24 hours) and sustained loss of LH receptors[118] was associated with increased serum LH, dysphasic serum FSH, decreased serum prolactin (PRL), a delay and reduction in the implantational surge of estradiol, and decreased serum progesterone.[121] From the chronology of these effects, the downregulatory property of LH, and the supportive role of PRL during this period in maintaining luteal LH receptors and luteal function, it was proposed that the disruption of ovarian steroidogenesis was a result of an LH:PRL imbalance.[122] The delay and attenuation of the pre-implantational estradiol surge and the reduced levels of progesterone were, in turn, responsible for the high incidence of implantational failure and, for those blastocysts that did implant, the steroidal milieu was inappropriate for their survival thereby leading to resorption. As with the pre-implantational LHRH treatment, post-implantational administration of LHRH and certain agonists has been found to produce a rapid and sustained reduction in luteal LH receptors.[118] This loss of luteal LH responsiveness is associated with progressively decreasing progesterone levels and failure of the pregnancy.[123] Similarly, administration of D-Ala^6-Des-Gly^{10}-Pro^9-NHEt-LHRH to regularly cycling female rats as a single injection on metestrus resulted in a marked depression in ovarian LH receptors within 1 day and reduced uterine weights and plasma progesterone as observed 2 days following the treatment.[120] Chronic treatment with this agonist led to significant reductions in ovarian LH, FSH and PRL receptor levels as well as in plasma progesterone and estradiol.[124]

While the reproductive dysfunction subsequent to LHRH or agonist treatment appears to take place mainly through the pituitary-gonadal axis, recent evidence has pointed to effects generated beyond the hypophysis. In pregnant rats, hypophysectomy on day 12 or 13 of gestation does not interfere with the viability of pregnancy, since the placenta assumes the role of the pituitary gland at this stage.[125,126] Administration of LHRH or agonists to such hypophysectomized-pregnant rats leads to pregnancy failure, implying a direct effect on either the ovary, the placenta or both.[127,128] The placenta has been investigated as a likely site for the extrapituitary effect in view of its importance in subserving the pituitary's role in supporting luteal function at this time. However, measurement of rat placental lactogen (rPL), a component of the placental luteotrophic complex, and serum progesterone, indicates that the anti-pregnancy mechanism of LHRH and its agonistic analogs in hypophysectomized rats involves an inhibition of luteal progesterone production which is reflected, but not initiated, by reduced rPL secretion. In fact, replacement with progesterone was able to reverse these effects (Fig. 5). The potential remaining extrapituitary sites through which these peptides might exert their inhibitory influence on progesterone secretion might include a direct ovarian action or by affecting placental hormones other than rPL necessary for luteal support. Relevant to this latter possibility are the observations that the human placenta synthesizes, stores and is responsive to LHRH.[129-131] The

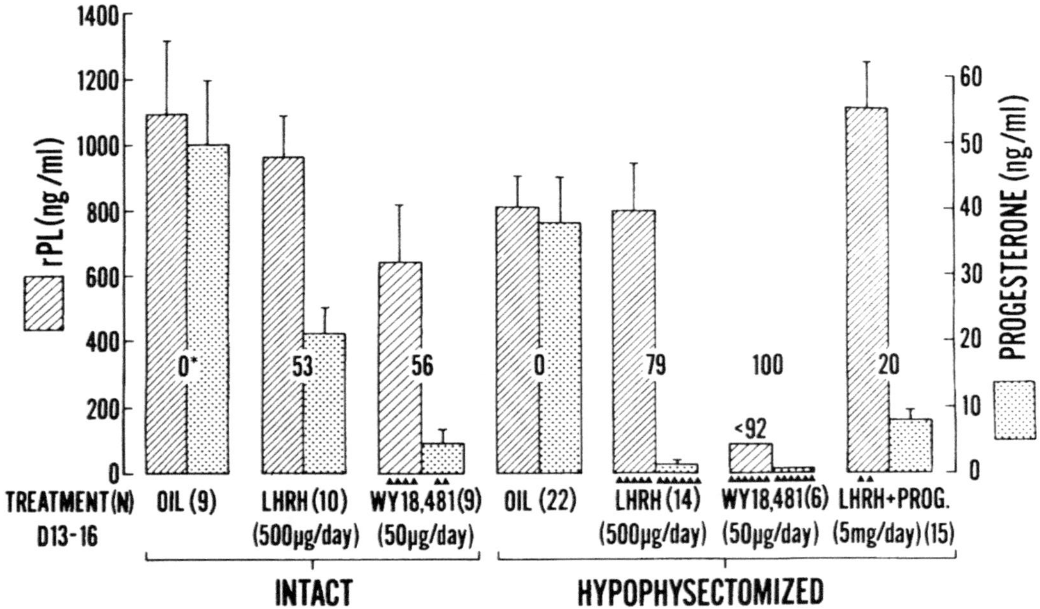

FIG. 5: Effect of treatment with LHRH or D-Ala^{6}-Des-Gly^{10}-Pro^{9}-NHEt-LHRH (Wy-18,481), on serum rat placental lactogen (rPL) and progesterone when administered to intact and hypophysectomized rats on days 13-16 of pregnancy. Hypophysectomy was performed on day 13 of pregnancy. Sacrifice and hormone determination was performed on day 18 of pregnancy. Individual animals with hormone values below the sensitivity of the respective assays are represented as Δ. The percentage of animals in which pregnancy was terminated by the various treatments are indicated within the graphical representation of each group's hormone levels (e.g. this value for the intact oil group is indicated by the *).

rat placental luteotropic complex has been indirectly identified as including, in addition to rPL, a putative LH-like chorionic gonadotropin[132] which presumably stimulates the luteal estradiol production necessary for a normal progesterone pattern.[133,134] However, there is rapidly increasing evidence that LHRH and the agonists can exert a direct action on the ovary. These studies have demonstrated that the LH-releasing peptides can: inhibit chorionic gonadotropin-induced ovarian and uterine weight gain in hypophysectomized rats and are competitively taken up by the ovary;[114,135] inhibit steroidogenesis induced by FSH in cultured granulosa cells from intact and hypophysectomized immature rats;[136] inhibit in vivo stimulation of ovarian function by FSH in hypophysectomized immature rats;[136] bind to isolated luteal cells from PMS + hCG-primed immature rats and inhibit in vitro production of progesterone by these cells;[137] inhibit follicular development and ovulation in PMS- or PMS + hCG-primed acutely hypophysectomized immature rats;[138] and locally inhibit pregnancy in rats following unilateral uterine instillation.[138a]

Although the release of inappropriately high levels of LH from the pituitary leading to a reduction in ovarian LH receptor content and a disruption of LH-dependent steroidogenesis would seem sufficient to explain the antifertility effects of LHRH and its agonistic analogs, it is quite apparent that a direct non-pituitary mechanism(s) is involved as well. However, the identification of specific gonadal LHRH/agonist binding and its effect on steroidogenesis present interesting questions, not only concerning the contribution of this process to the antifertility activity of rather large exogenous doses of LHRH and its agonists, but the function of this binding in the normal reproductive process; particularly, since peripheral endogenous levels of LHRH are extremely low. Clayton[137] suggests that possibly LHRH or a related peptide might be synthesized in the uterus (placenta?) or in the ovary where it might serve locally as a mediator of luteolysis. This concept takes on additional significance in view of the observations that the human placenta synthesizes and stores a peptide with immunological and biological LHRH-like activity.

c) Reversibility of antifertility effects in the female

It was of critical importance to the further development of the LHRH agonist contraceptive utility that the effects be specific and reversible. Safety studies including ancillary pharmacology and preliminary toxicologic evaluation will be considered in a separate section. The restoration of fertility following both pre- and post-coital administration has received much attention. The vaginal smear type of rats receiving LHRH/agonist treatment before and after implantation were found to change by midgestation from a leucocytic smear characteristic of pregnancy to one which was predominantly cornified.[106,139] Confirmation that this break in smear type represented pregnancy termination and a resumption of cyclicity was provided by the fact that all animals exposed to males during this post-treatment segment mated and carried to normal, uneventful term. While 4-or 8-day pre-coital administration with LHRH or a potent LHRH agonist delays the appearance of expected estrus and mating, and reduces the fertility of those that do mate, regular cyclicity is re-established within one week following termination of treatment.[112] Supportive evidence for a direct relationship between the total dose of the LH-releasing peptide administered (irrespective of route) and the length of time required for resumption of cyclicity is provided in Figure 6 where D-Trp^{6}-N-MeLeu^{7}-Des-Gly^{10}-Pro^{9}-NHEt-LHRH (Wy-40,972) was utilized as a representative agonist. It is particularly interesting that not only is there a linear relationship between the return interval and the total dose administered, but that the slope is shallow with large increases in dose only minimally prolonging the acyclic period. These results indicate the reversibility of the inhibitory effects of Wy-40,972 on reproductive function, and are in agreement with those of Johnson et al.[115] who demonstrated that daily treatment with 100 μg/kg, sc of the potent LHRH agonist, D-Leu^{6}-Des-Gly^{10}-Pro^{9}-NHEt-LHRH, for 77 days was followed, within 20 days after the termination of treatment, by successful mating resulting in the birth of normally sized litters of healthy pups.

d) Studies in women and future prospectives

The plethora of animal data in both sexes has clearly defined the nature of and reasons why this genre of compound now appears to represent, specifically in the female, one of the major advances in contraceptive development since the advent of the steroidal oral contraceptives. Extension of the anti-reproductive animal data into the clinic has led to several investigations demonstrating the luteolytic and emmenagogic properties of LHRH and selected agonists. Quite appropriately and predictably, the doses chosen were based on the LH-releasing property of the compounds, the criterion that was previously employed in the attempted pro-fertility approach. The LH-releasing doses of various agonists in human females and males and their routes of administration

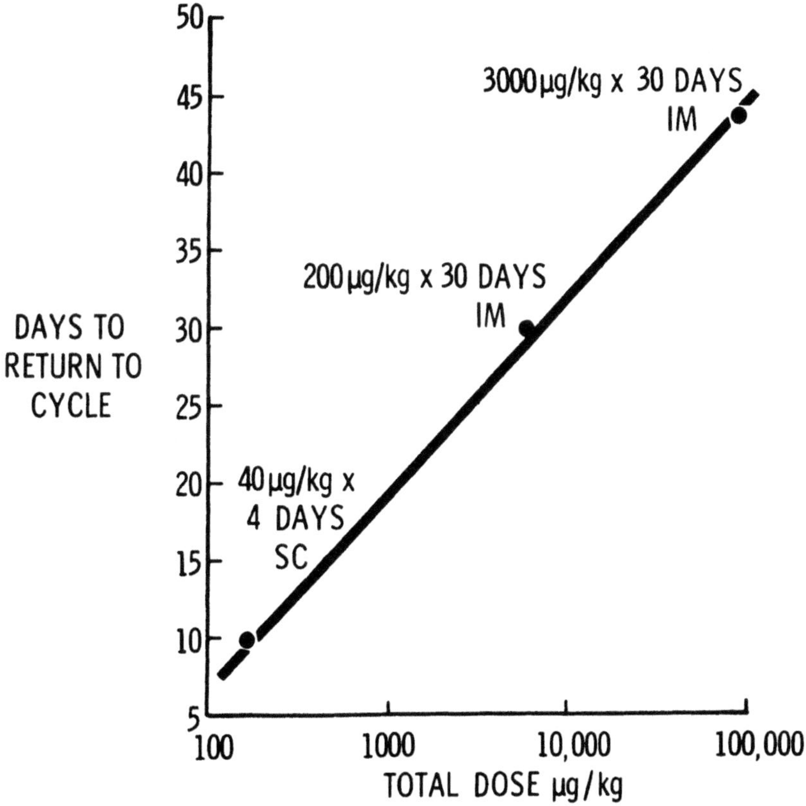

FIG. 6: Return to estrous cyclicity in rats treated with D-Trp^{6}-N-MeLeu^{7}-Des-Gly^{10}-Pro^{9}-NHEt-LHRH (Wy-40,972).

are depicted in Table 5. It was initially observed that with a total of 1250 μg LHRH administered subcutaneously as a divided dose at 4-hour intervals over a 20-hour period starting between 1 to 9 days following ovulation, the luteal phase was shortened between 1 and 4 days and progesterone levels were reduced to half that observed in the control subjects.[43] Supporting the direct relationship between agonist (LH-releasing activity) and antifertility potency established in laboratory animals, only 100 μg of a superagonist (D-Trp^6-Des-Gly^{10}-Pro^9-NHEt-LHRH) given in divided doses, subcutaneously (sc), on 2 days during the midluteal phase[44] or a total of 500 μg of another agonist (Des-Gly^{10}-Pro^9-NHEt-LHRH) given in 5 daily injections (sc) during the early luteal phase[42] was capable of a similar luteolytic and emmenagogic effect. Intranasal dosages of 1 mg of D-$Ser(TBu)^6$-Des-Gly^{10}-Pro^9-NHEt-LHRH (Buserelin®) administered on days 4-9 following the midcycle LH peak also decreased progesterone and shortened the cycle.[140] The two cycles following cessation of this treatment were considered to be normal and ovulatory in nature. Daily administration (sc) with a 5 μg dose of Buserelin® during an entire menstrual cycle was found to inhibit ovulation as well as the expected luteal progesterone increase and the subsequent non-treatment cycle was found to be normal.[41] Similar chronic treatment extended for up to 12 weeks consistently inhibited ovulation and resulted in insufficient luteal phases. It was particularly encouraging that chronic intranasal administration of this agonist for up to 180 days (600 μg/day),[45,141] which produced anovulatory cycles, did not generally affect normal menstrual bleeding. In all of these chronic treatment studies, normal ovulatory cycles returned within an average of one month following termination of treatment.

Extensive trials are now required to establish contraceptive acceptability related to unprotected intercourse. Based on the post-coital pregnancy-terminating

TABLE 5

EFFECT OF LH-RH AND AGONISTS ON LH RELEASE IN MAN BY VARIOUS ROUTES OF ADMINISTRATION

COMPOUND	SC	IM	PO	NASAL (Drops or Spray)	VAGINAL	RECTAL
	LH-RELEASING DOSE, µg/PERSON					
LH-RH	100-250	25	--	500; 1200-1300	--	--
D-Leu^{6}-DesGly^{10}-Pro^{9}-NHEt-LH-RH	5-25	5-10	10,000	100	2000	2000
D-Trp^{6}-DesGly^{10}-Pro^{9}-NHEt-LH-RH	10	10	--	50;~500	--	--
D-Ser(TBU)^{6}-DesGly^{10}-Pro^{9}-NHEt-LH-RH (Buserelin)	5	--	--	>200<400 (ointment) 10-100	--	--
D-Trp^{6}-LH-RH	10	10	--	500	--	--
D-Ala^{6}-DesGly^{10}-Pro^{9}-NHEt-LH-RH	--	150	--	500	--	--
D-Phe^{6}-DesGly^{10}-Pro^{9}-NHEt-LH-RH	--	--	--	500	--	--

studies in animals, late luteal and early pregnancy (4-6 weeks of gestation) regimens also would be appropriate. In this regard, it will be interesting to determine whether the peptides will be effective when support for pregnancy has shifted to placental production of hCG and other hormones. Quite possibly the presence of direct placental/ovarian effects, as identified in laboratory studies, could become crucial for their activity in this particular contraceptive application.

Thus, it is quite clear that the antifertility properties of this class of peptides, first identified in laboratory animals, are not only evident in humans but present much promise as fertility-regulating agents. Moreover, the human studies verify the direct relationship between LH-releasing activity and luteolysis which, in turn, provides a valuable predictive basis for developing this particular contraceptive approach.

2. Antifertility Potential in the Male

a) Effects on male reproductive function

Examination of potential LHRH- and agonist-induced antifertility effects in the male became the subject of intense interest, particularly on the basis of their anti-reproductive properties in the female and the general inability of these compounds to significantly ameliorate various types of clinical andropathy (hypospermia, hypogonadotropic hypogonadism, etc.). In the male, as in the female, LH and hCG have been shown to negatively affect gonadal LH receptor concentrations;[142,143] in view of the established role of LH-induced LH receptor downregulation in the antifertility effects of LHRH and its agonists in the female, the former have provided further support for their possible disruptive influence on male reproductive processes. Subsequently, numerous laboratory studies confirmed this presumptive evidence and directly identified a variety of anti-reproductive effects produced by this class of peptide in the male which included: weight loss of the testes, seminal vesicles and ventral prostate, histologic disruption of spermatogonia, seminiferous tubules and Sertoli cells, decreased spermatogenesis and testosterone production, and decreased incidence of mating and fertility.[40,139,144-149] These results have not only corroborated the predominantly antifertility profile of these compounds elucidated in the female and provided some explanation for the equivocal results obtained from their attempted therapeutic clinical application but allude to the possibility that LHRH/agonists may represent a novel and much sought-after approach to male fertility regulation.

Initial studies in the rat employing such potent LHRH agonists as D-Leu^{6}-Des-Gly^{10}-Pro^{9}-NHEt-LHRH and D-Ala^{6}-Des-Gly^{10}-Pro^{9}-NHEt-LHRH at daily dosages greater than 1 μg demonstrated that significant depression in the weights of the testes and in peripheral testosterone concentrations could be obtained within one week of treatment.[139,144,145,147] Further evaluation revealed that not only were much lower dosages capable of producing effects of a similar magnitude and that the weights of the seminal vesicles and ventral prostate were also reduced but that continued treatment resulted in a progressive disorganization of the seminiferous tubules, loss of sperm in the tubular lumina and loss of staining characteristics of spermatogonia and of interstitial cells.[40,139,144,148,149-151] However, from a standpoint of prospective contraceptive utility, it was apparent that the chronology of these effects presented an inappropriate dissociation. In other words, the desired effects on spermatogenesis and fertility were found to be consistently associated with, and generally preceded by, marked depression in reproductive organ weights and a reduction in mating behavior. A variety of agonistic analogs, dosages, and treatment schedules have been employed unsuccessfully in attempts to desynchronize the spermatogenic process and/or disrupt epididymal maturation without affecting other testosterone-dependent targets. In this regard, administration of 0.1 μg D-Ala^6-Des-Gly^{10}-Pro^9-NHEt-LHRH as infrequently as once weekly for 11 weeks, representing approximately 1.5 rat spermatogenic cycles, significantly reduced reproductive organ weights without affecting mating performance or fertility.[139]

While various short-term regimens with LHRH treatment have been found to be sufficient to negatively affect the steroidal milieu necessary for the series of discrete events involved in female reproduction (i.e. ovulation, implantation), in the male, where gametogenesis is a continually renewing and overlapping process, chronic suppression of testicular function appears necessary to inhibit fertility. Considering the evidence that such treatment would also be associated with adverse and quite possibly irreversible effects on other androgen-dependent organs as well as sexual behavior, it seems that the desired effect (i.e. a "pharmacologic vasectomy") will be difficult to obtain with the LH-releasing peptides; this situation is not unlike that encountered with the attempted use of various steroids and their combinations to develop a chemical male contraceptive. Since the LH-releasing peptides present a predominantly anti-reproductive pharmacologic profile in the male and, as in the female, the severity of these effects are directly related to their potency, dosage, and dosing frequency, current efforts to achieve successful treatments for hypogonadotropic hypogonadism, oligospermia, delayed puberty or cryptorchidism, through the development of more potent and long-acting LHRH agonists, should be reconsidered. Regarding the latter two clinical applications, chronic treatment of immature male rats with LHRH or various agonists has been shown, depending on dose and length of administration, to retard growth of the testes, seminal vesicles and ventral prostate, depress serum testosterone levels and disrupt testicular histology.[144,152-155]

b) Mechanism of anti-reproductive effects in the male

On the basis of the identification of an LHRH/agonist-induced LH-receptor loss in the female, its association with inappropriately elevated endogenous LH levels, and the ability of LH and hCG to reduce testicular LH receptors, the observation that the LH-releasing peptides could initiate a similar downregulatory phenomenon in the male, resulting in a marked and prolonged loss in LH receptors, was not entirely unexpected.[139,144-146] However, it was particularly interesting that dosages of the agonists that had minimal effects on reproductive organ weights were also found to depress LH receptor binding.[139,145,146] Although it was possible that the depressed binding in these instances might be due to receptor occupancy, inhibition of this parameter was generally associated with lowered LH-dependent steroidogenesis. Thus, it might be suggested that the reduction in reproductive organ weights produced by higher dosages of the agonist occur through processes in addition to inhibition of LH binding. In this regard, it has been recently demonstrated that a single administration of LHRH can induce a loss in testicular FSH and PRL receptor sites but this effect required higher dosages than those producing effects on LH binding and testosterone production.[156] Although it might be speculated that the effect of LHRH on FSH and PRL receptors occurs through alterations in pituitary secretion of these hormones leading to the loss of required positive support (possibly PRL)[157] or, as demonstrated for LH, initiation of a downregulatory process (possibly FSH), it has become increasingly apparent that direct, non-pituitary mediated effects of the LHRH/agonists on gonadal receptors and/or steroidogenesis may be involved as well.

Recent studies utilizing immature male rats demonstrated that LHRH can inhibit FSH-induced increases in testicular function either _in vitro_ or in hypophysectomized animals *in vivo* and reduce binding of hCG to Leydig cells in both FSH-treated and untreated immature hypophysectomized rats.[158] Additionally, a potent LHRH agonist has been shown to accelerate atrophy of the testes and sex accessory organs in hypophysectomized immature rats.[139,144] However, elaboration of a similar extrapituitary profile in the adult male has been less clear. It has been reported that adult rat testes will specifically bind D-Trp^6-LHRH, and that this agonist as well as D-Ser(TBu)^6-Des-Gly^{10}-Pro^9-NHEt-LHRH produce in hypophysectomized male rats, a reduction in testicular LH receptors and accumulation of steroidogenic intermediates prior to testosterone.[159,160] However, it was also reported that regression of the testes and sex accessory organ weights of hypophysectomized adult male rats occurred at the same rate whether or not they had been treated for an extended period with large doses of a potent LHRH agonist, D-Ala^6-Des-Gly^{10}-Pro^9-NHEt-LHRH.[139] *In vitro* incubation of testicular homogenates from intact adult rats with either D-Trp^6- or D-Ala^6-Des-Gly^{10}-Pro^9-NHEt-LHRH did not affect basal or hCG-stimulated steroidogenesis, whereas *in vivo* administration of either peptide prior to the *in vitro* test did depress testosterone production.[139,161] However, when hypophysectomized adult males were given similar *in vivo* exposure to D-Ala^6-Des-Gly^{10}-Pro^9-NHEt-LHRH there was no measurable affect on steroidogenic response *in vitro* when compared with testes from control hypophysectomized rats.[139] Moreover, concurrent administration of testosterone propionate, which was unable to completely reverse the inhibition of testicular weights and seminiferous tubule morphology induced by D-Trp^6-Des-Gly^{10}-Pro^9-NHEt-LHRH in intact males, was capable of maintaining qualitatively normal spermatogenesis in hypophysectomized agonist-treated rats.[149]

Thus, while it appears in the adult male that a pituitary-mediated mechanism plays an important role in the antifertility properties of LHRH and its agonists, the nature and extent of the contribution to these effects of a possible direct gonadal action(s) is as yet unclear.

Pituitary "exhaustion" or refractoriness to continued stimulation by LHRH or the agonists might represent another component in the mechanism by which reproductive collapse is induced or at least exacerbated by these peptides. In this regard, the LH response of cultured pituitary cells was attenuated by chronic exposure to D-Trp^{6}-Des-Gly^{10}-Pro^{9}-NHEt-LHRH[149] and chronic administration of D-$Ser(TBu)^{6}$-Des-Gly^{10}-Pro^{9}-NHEt-LHRH to castrated male rats resulted in reduced plasma and pituitary gonadotropin content.[157]

The marked LHRH/agonist-induced inhibition of testosterone production, possibly occurring as a result of the pituitary-mediated and/or direct gonadal effects discussed previously, is characterized by a block in the steroidogenic pathway at the 17-hydroxylase and 17,20-desmolase level.[162,163] This leads to the accumulation of testosterone precursors, most notably evidenced by increases in plasma progesterone.[149,164] Progesterone elevation, in view of its inhibitory effects on spermatogenesis in the rat[165] has, in fact, been suggested to contribute to the antigonadal effects of LHRH and the agonists.[149,164] Moreover, the presumed increase in testicular 5^{α}-reductase and possibly aromatose activity, in response to LHRH or D-Ala^{6}-Des-Gly^{10}-Pro^{9}-NHEt-LHRH, and resulting in the maintenance of relatively normal DHT and estradiol levels, might further aggravate the testosterone depletion.[152,163]

c) Reversibility of antifertility effects in the male

The effects of a potential chemical contraceptive should be completely reversible and the male's reproductive processes should return to normalcy following cessation of treatment within a reasonable period of time. In a recent study where the inhibitory effects of a potent agonist, D-Ala^{6}-Des-Gly^{10}-Pro^{9}-NHEt-LHRH, on male rat reproduction were maximized by administering

1 mg daily for 35 days, it was demonstrated that both testicular LH binding and serum testosterone had significantly rebounded by day 14, post-treatment, and approximated control values by day 44.[144] Restoration of breeding processes became evident between days 14-28 post-treatment and were fully restored by day 44. Although testicular histologic repair and functional recrudescence appeared generally normal by days 14-28 post-treatment, small degenerative or calcified areas still were observable at day 70. The weights of the testes, possibly reflecting the histological background picture, were still somewhat depressed, as were the weights of the seminal vesicles and ventral prostate. However, all of these organs' weights revealed a growth pattern similar to, but more rapid than that of controls; any initial differences became insignificant with time. Much lower dosages, 5 μg, of an agonist of similar potency, D-Trp^6-Des-Gly^{10}-Pro^9-NHEt-LHRH, when administered for one week, resulted in qualitatively similar inhibitory effects;[149,164] (it should be noted that the effects of the 1 mg/day treatment with the D-Ala^6-analog are maximal within 14 days and that a similar degree of inhibition can be obtained with daily dosages of 1 μg).[139] Seminal vesicle weights and testosterone levels had returned to control values one week after terminating treatment. While testes weights had rebounded significantly at one week post-treatment they were still only 80% of the controls at 4 weeks. Particularly significant was the observation that 30-40% of the tubules were exhibiting disrupted germinal epithelium at 4 weeks post-treatment. In general, it might be stated that cessation of agonist treatment is followed by a differential restoration of affected targets whose chronology is dependent on the dose of the agonist and its duration of administration. However, in view of the projected necessity for chronic administration of these peptides for male contraceptive application, it is particularly important that more

information be obtained concerning the capability and the length of time required to achieve complete restoration.

d) Future prospectives for LHRH agonists as male contraceptives

Consideration of LHRH/agonists as possible male contraceptive agents has and still is, based primarily on laboratory results (vide supra) and indirectly by their inability to correct various andropathic disorders and the identification that their subacute administration in males leads to reduced gonadotropin responses.[57,58] However, the gametogenic pattern in the male, in contrast to the female, is a protracted, qualitatively and quantitatively complicated series of continuous events. While a variety of short-term strategies serve to regulate fertility in the female (e.g. neuroendocrine ovulatory blockade, induction of luteolysis, inhibition or interference with nidatory events), the constantly renewing and overlapping waves of spermatogenic development have generally limited the search for a male antifertility agent to chronic approaches. Long-term (17 weeks) daily administration of 5 µg D-Ser(TBu)^{6}-Des-Gly^{10}-Pro^{9}-NHEt-LHRH to normal men, to specifically assess the antifertility effects of this treatment, revealed a significant reduction in basal serum gonadotropin and testosterone levels which was reversed within one week after the termination of treatment.[59] However, this dosing regimen, which was found to inhibit ovulation in normally ovulating women,[41] did not affect spermatogenesis or potency. While chronic schedules utilizing higher dosages may lead to inhibition of sperm production, the further retardation of androgen secretion can lead to problems of impotency and potential atrophy of secondary sexual accessory tissues, as have been observed in animal studies. Because the nature of the spermatogenic cycle dictates chronic pharmacologic intervention, which has been found to produce an inappropriate dissociation between spermatogenesis and androgen production, use of the agonists as a male contraceptive has been confronted with many obstacles, not unlike those seen in an attempt to develop a steroidal male contraceptive; thus, at this time, the LHRH agonists do not appear to represent a viable approach to male fertility regulation. However, the observation by Rivier _et al._[149] that administration of testosterone concurrently with a potent agonist was able to significantly restore the weights of the testes and sex accessory organs without reversing the agonist-induced tubular degeneration and inhibition of mitotic activity, allude to the possibility that with appropriate supplemental steroidal support, the agonists eventually might be used to selectively inhibit spermatogenesis. However, the advantage of this approach over steroid-only methods presently being evaluated are debatable. Moreover, the problems which would be encountered in determining efficacious and safe dosages and dosing regimens for agonist-steroid combinations seem monumental.

3. Safety Studies: Secondary Pharmacology and Preliminary Toxicologic Evaluation

LHRH and several agonists have been subjected to a battery of tests to determine their toxicologic liability and their potential effects on non-reproductive organ systems in rats. The results of a preliminary acute intravenous toxicologic study and associated effects on the central nervous system in mature female rats are described in Table 6. It is to be noted that the dosages required to produce these untoward effects are in considerable excess of those required for the primary agonist (ovulation induction) effect.

A more extensive evaluation, seen in Table 7, relates the reproductive pharmacologic effects of D-Trp^{6}-N-MeLeu^{7}-Des-Gly^{10}-Pro^{9}-NHEt-LHRH (Wy-40,972) to those observed in ancillary (non-reproductive) tests. It is quite apparent that under proposed and realistic clinical dosing regimens anticipated for

TABLE 6

PRELIMINARY ACUTE TOXICOLOGY OF LHRH AGONISTS IN MATURE FEMALE RATS

COMPOUND	N	DOSE TESTED μg/kg, I.V.	% LETHALITY	REMARKS	AGONIST (OVULATION INDUCING) DOSE MED 100* μg/kg, I.V.
LHRH	5	50,000	0	SLIGHT ATAXIA.	>8<40
WY-18,186 (D-Ala^6-LHRH)	5	400	0	ALL RATS APPEARED NORMAL.	4.0
WY-18,481 (D-Ala^6-DesGly^{10}-Pro^9-NHEt-LHRH)	3	50,000	33	ATAXIA, RESPIRATORY DEPRESSION, LOSS OF MUSCLE TONE, LOSS OF GRASPING AND RIGHTING REFLEXES, CYANOSIS. DEATH WITHIN 9 MIN.	4.0
WY-40,972 (D-Trp^6-N-MeLeu^7-DesGly^{10}-Pro^9-NHEt-LHRH)	3	5,000	0	ALL RATS APPEARED NORMAL.	0.40
	3	10,000	100	REDUCED MOTOR ACTIVITY, DEPRESSION, ATAXIA, RESPIRATORY DISTRESS. DEATH WITHIN 7 MIN.	

*Approximate minimal effective 100% dose.

TABLE 7

GENERAL PHARMACOLOGIC PROFILE OF WY-40,972 IN RAT

REPRODUCTIVE PHARMACOLOGY						ANCILLARY PHARMACOLOGY						
OVULATION INDUCTION		LH RELEASE	POST-COITAL CONTRACEPTION			CNS GENERAL		GI: GASTRIC ACID SECRETION	GI: MOTILITY		CV: BLOOD PRESSURE/HEART RATE	RENAL
TOTAL ED_{100}* µg/kg						TOTAL DOSE µg/kg++						
IV	PO	IV	SC	IM	PO	IP	IV	SC	SC	PO	IM	PO
0.40+	40+	.004+	28‡	400+ 280‡	5600-24000‡	1,000 (STIMULATION, IRRITATION)	> 5,000 <10,000 GENERAL DEPRESSION AND DEATH	NO EFFECT AT 1,000	NO EFFECT AT 10,000		SLIGHT AND TRANSIENT INCREASE AT 1000	NO DIURETIC EFFECT AT 100,000

*ED_{100} Approximate minimum 100% effective dose
+ As single administration
‡ As multiple administration
++ Approximate minimum effective dose

their utilitarian (contraceptive) application there would be a large margin of safety.

The inhibition and recovery of the reproductive organs observed following sub-acute, high dose studies, and related acceptable safety margins have been demonstrated with LHRH[106,166] and several related agonists: D-Leu^{6}-Des-Gly^{10}-Pro^{9}-NHEt-LHRH,[113] D-Ala^{6}-Des-Gly^{10}-Pro^{9}-NHEt-LHRH,[40,106,139,144] D-Ser(TBu)^{6}-Des-Gly^{10}-Pro^{9}-NHEt-LHRH[167] and D-Trp^{6}-Des-Gly^{10}-Pro^{9}-NHEt-LHRH.[149] Furthermore, other investigations have indicated the lack of teratogenic liability for compounds of this type.[168] Collectively, the data in the literature have demonstrated that this class of compound is well-tolerated and provides a wide and highly acceptable therapeutic ratio both in animal[169-171] and in chronic human investigations.[41,45,141]

IV. CONCLUSIONS

The past nine years have borne witness to dramatic advances in the development of the chemistry and pharmacology of LHRH and its peptidic analogues. Approximately 1000 compounds have been synthesized and evaluated for potential use as contraceptive agents, based on either their ability to inhibit gonadotropin secretion and consequently, ovulation, or to produce paradoxical antifertility effects in pregnant and non-pregnant animal models. The former class encompasses the LHRH antagonists, the latter, the LHRH ("super") agonists. Historically, the LHRH antagonists represented the first subclass to be synthesized and biologically identified, based on the premise that such inhibitory analogues would prevent the secretion of LH and of FSH, thereby blocking ovulation. However, both the animal and meager clinical investigations with the most potent of these compounds have demonstrated the necessity for relatively high doses given by restricted and hence, potentially impractical dosing regimens to produce anti-ovulatory effects. To date, while research continues in this area and the recent identification of certain extremely potent antagonists might improve prospects for their future application, the most promising developments (in terms of scope of animal and clinical investigations) have occurred with the agonists. In addition to their diagnostic utility, these compounds have been used extensively in attempts to therapeutically alter a wide spectrum of gynecopathic and andropathic conditions. While these agents clearly produce gonadotropin release, their effectiveness in inducing ovulation (and establishing subsequent pregnancy), normalizing amenorrheic states, hypogonadism, hypospermia, retarded puberty, etc., have been without significant reward. In fact, it was originally hoped that the availability of the more potent agonists would overcome the difficulties encountered with the parent molecule, LHRH, based on the synthesis of a generation of LHRH congeners that would possess, in addition to greater potency, prolonged duration of activity, greater receptor binding proper and increased resistance to enzymatic degradation. While these chemical and pharmacologic criteria have been fulfilled, the traditional pro-fertility application of these compounds still was encountered with frustration and disappointment. For years, it was presumed that these peptides would be useful fertility-inducing agents only if proper and carefully timed dosing regimens could be established.

However, it has become firmly established that the LH-releasing class of peptides possesses an essentially anti-reproductive pharmacologic profile which, rather than representing a contradiction of the integral role the parent molecule plays in normal reproductive function, reflects the complex pharmacologic nature of these peptides and the processes that they control. Notably, the recent identification of receptor downregulation by inappropriately elevated LH levels, as well as the extrapituitary actions of LHRH and its agonists, have contributed much to resolving the paradoxical pro-/ antifertility classification of these peptides. Moreover, extensive reproductive evaluation has consistently supported the potential of these substances for use as contraceptive agents in the female. In fact, short-term administration of several of these compounds to women during early and mid-segments of the luteal phase has been demonstrated to produce rapid luteolysis, progesterone decline and the premature onset of menses. This post-ovulatory luteal phase approach to potential contraception has been complemented with drug administration over an entire menstrual cycle, leading to inhibition of ovulation, shortened luteal phase and subsequent menstruation. Following withdrawal of treatment, normal ovulatory cycles return. Many of these studies have utilized a nasal spray mode of drug delivery thus providing a simple and practical means of administration.

The paradoxical antifertility effects of LHRH and agonists in the male corroborate those in the female, and perhaps explain, as has been offered for the female, the inability of such peptides to perform as efficacious pro-fertility agents. Specifically, the antifertility effects observed in the male subjected to LHRH agonist manipulation allude to the possibility that use of such peptides may represent a novel approach to male fertility regulation. However, while these agents do produce profound anti-reproductive effects in the male, including the desired inhibition of spermatogenesis and fertility, concomitant effects on the testes, sex accessory organs and libido must be minimized or completely eliminated before such an approach could be seriously considered.

The spectrum of reproductive effects and the toxicologic, pathologic and ancillary pharmacologic studies (e.g. CNS, gastrointestinal, cardiovascular, pulmonary, renal), involving varied dosing regimens and routes of administration have demonstrated the safety of selected LHRH agonists. Any undesirable side effects thus far noted in any of the animal models employed for safety evaluation have occurred at doses far exceeding those necessary for practical and utilitarian purposes. As such, these compounds present a therapeutic margin (contraceptive dose vs. dose producing untoward side effects) of considerable magnitude in laboratory studies. The long clinical record of safe, if relatively ineffective use as pro-fertility agents, and a rapidly increasing body of evidence for promising contraceptive utility, unencumbered by side effects, is most encouraging.

The collective animal and clinical data on the LHRH agonists have established their antifertility activity and, coupled with their demonstrated potency, reproducible efficacy, lack of significant secondary (non-reproductive) pharmacologic effects and no apparent compromise to safety under clinically realistic dosing protocols, clearly support their candidacy as potential contraceptives specifically in the female.

REFERENCES

1. Schally, A.V., Arimura, A., Baba, Y., Nair, R.M.G., Matsuo, H., Redding, T.W., Debeljuk, L., and White, W.F., Isolation and properties of the FSH and LH-releasing hormone, Biochem. Biophys. Res. Commun., 43, 393, 1971.

2. Schally, A.V., Nair, R.M.G., Redding, T.W., and Arimura, A., Isolation of the LH and FSH releasing hormone from porcine hypothalami , J. Biol. Chem., 246, 7230, 1971.

3. Matsuo, H., Baba, Y., Nair, R.M.G., Arimura, A., and Schally, A.V., Structure of the porcine LH and FSH releasing hormone. I. The proposed amino acid sequence, Biochem. Biophys. Res. Commun., 43, 1334, 1971.

4. Matsuo, H., Arimura, A., Nair, R.M.G., and Schally, A.V., Synthesis of the porcine LH and FSH releasing hormone by the solid phase method, Biochem. Biophys. Res. Commun., 45, 822, 1971.

5. Kastin, A.J., Schally, A.V., Gual, C., Midgley, A.R., Bowers, C.Y., and Diaz-Infante, A., Stimulation of LH release in men and women by hypothalamic LH-releasing hormone purified from porcine hypothalami , J. Clin. Endocrinol. Metab., 29, 1046, 1969.

6. Kastin, A.V., Schally, A.V., Gual, C., Midgley, A.R., Bowers, C.Y., and Gomez-Perez, E., Administration of LH-releasing hormone to selected human subjects, Am. J. Obstet. Gynecol., 108, 177, 1970.

7. Kastin, A.J., Zarate, A., Midgley, A.R., Canales, E.S., and Schally, A.V., Ovulation confirmed by pregnancy after infusion of porcine LH-RH, J. Clin. Endocrinol. Metab., 33, 980, 1971.

8. Taymor, M.L., The use of luteinizing hormone-releasing hormone in gynecologic endocrinology, Fertil. Steril., 25, 992, 1974.

9. Zarate, A., Canales, E.S., Soria, J., Forsbach, G., Kastin, A.J., and Schally, A.V., Therapeutic use of gonadoliberin (follicle-stimulating

hormone/luteinizing hormone-releasing hormone) in women, Fertil. Steril., 27, 1233, 1976.

10. Akande, E.O., Carr, P.J., Dutton, A., Bonnar, J., Corker, C.S., McKinnon, P.C.B., and Robinson, D., Effect of synthetic gonadotrophin releasing hormone in secondary amenorrhea, Lancet, 2, 112, 1972.

11. Keller, P.J., Induction of ovulation by synthetic luteinizing hormone releasing factor in infertile women, Lancet, 2, 570, 1972.

12. Keller, P.J., Treatment of anovulation with synthetic luteinizing hormone releasing hormone, Am. J. Obstet. Gynecol., 116, 698, 1973.

13. Bonnar, J.J., Studies in the use of luteinizing hormone-follicle-stimulating hormone releasing hormone to induce ovulation in women, J. Endocrinol., 58, xxxiv, 1973.

14. Breckwoldt, M., Czygan, P.-J., Lehmann, F., and Bettendorf, G., Synthetic LH-RH as a therapeutic agent, Acta Endocrinol., 75, 209, 1974.

15. Nakano, R., Katayama, K., Mizuno, T., and Tojo, S., Induction of ovulation with synthetic luteinizing hormone-releasing hormone, Fertil. Steril., 25, 471, 1974.

16. Pedersen, P.H., Larsen, J.F., Micic, S., Roos, J., and Sele, V., The effects of intravenous synthetic luteinizing hormone releasing hormone (LHRH) in infertile women with anovulation, Acta Obstet. Gynecol. Scand., 53, 89, 1974.

17. Zarate, A., Canales, E.S., Soria, J., Gonzalez, A., Schally, A.V., and Kastin, A.J., Further observations on the therapy of anovulatory infertility with synthetic luteinizing hormone-releasing hormone, Fertil. Steril., 25, 3, 1974.

18. Zanartu, J., Dabancens, A., Kastin, A.J., and Schally, A.V., Effect of synthetic hypothalamic gonadotropin-releasing hormone (FSH/LH-RH) in anovulatory sterility, Fertil. Steril., 25, 160, 1974.

19. Figueroa Casas, P.R., Badano, A.R., Aparicio, N., Lencioni, L.J., Berli, R.R., Badano, H., Biccoca, C., and Schally, A.V., Luteinizing hormone-releasing hormone in the treatment of anovulatory infertility, Fertil. Steril., 26, 549, 1975.

20. Zanartu, J., Dabancens, A., Rodriguez-Bravo, R., Barsby, F., and Schally, A.V., Ovulation induction: Ovarian response to human gonadotropins and synthetic gonadotropin-releasing hormone, Obstet. Gynecol., 45, 443, 1975.

21. Henderson, S.R., Bonnar, J., Moore, A., and MacKinnon, P., Luteinizing hormone-releasing hormone for induction of follicular maturation and ovulation in women with infertility and amenorrhea, Fertil. Steril., 27, 621, 1976.

22. Huang, K.E., Use of synthetic luteinizing hormone-releasing hormone in induction of ovulation in amenorrheic patients, Fertil. Steril., 26, 796, 1975.

23. Figueroa Casas, P.R., Miechi, H., Badano, A., Mirkin, A., Aparicio, N., Turner, D., Nagle, C., and Rosner, J., Clinical and gonadotropic response of amenorrheic patients treated with clomiphene and repeated injections of luteinizing hormone-releasing hormone, Fertil. Steril., 28, 293, 1977.

24. Bohnet, H.G., Dahlan, H.G., Keller, E., Friedrich, F., Schindler, A.E., Wyss, H.I., Schneider, H.P.G., Human pituitary gonadotropin index. II. LH-RH test and clomiphene response before and after LH-RH stimulation, Clin. Endocrinol., 5, 25, 1976.

25. Schally, A.V., Kastin, A.J., and Coy, D.H., LH-releasing hormone and its analogues: Recent basic and clinical investigations, Int. J. Fertil., 21, 1, 1976.

26. Vale, W., Rivier, C., and Brown, M., Regulatory peptides of the hypothalamus, Ann. Rev. Physiol., 39, 473, 1977.

27. Schally, A.V., Coy, D.H., and Meyers, C.A., Hypothalamic regulatory hormones, Ann. Rev. Biochem., 47, 89, 1978.

28. de Medeiros-Comaru, A.M., Rodriguez, J., Povoa, L.C., Franco, S., Dimetz, T., Coy, D.H., Kastin, A.J., and Schally, A.V., Clinical studies with long-acting superactive analogs of LH-RH in women with secondary amenorrhea, Int. J. Fertil., 21, 239, 1976.

29. Cortes-Prieto, J., Arenciba-Rocha, J., Aranda, A., Garcia-Garcia, Ma.-D., Coy, D.H., and Schally, A.V., Attempts to induce ovulation in amenorrheic patients using D-Ala-6-LH-RH propylamide, Int. J. Fertil., 24, 108, 1977.

30. Nillius, S.J., and Wide, L., Acute and chronic effects of the stimulatory luteinizing hormone-releasing hormone analogue D-SER(TBU)^{6}-EA^{10}-LRH on the gonadotrophin and gonadal steroid secretion in women with amenorrhea, Acta Endocrinol., Suppl. 212, 138, 1977.

31. Hanker, J.P., Bohnet, H.G., Mühlenstedt, D., Nowack, C., and Schneider, H.P.G., Gonadotrophin release during chronic administration of D-Ser(TBU)^{6} LH-RH-EA in functional amenorrhea, Acta Endocrinol., 89, 625, 1978.

32. Botella-Llusia, A.J., Jaramillo, C., and Charro-Salgado, A., Trial of a new analogue of LH-RH in normal subjects and in cases of anovulatory sterility, Acta Obstet. Gynecol. Scand., 56, 337, 1977.

33. Jaramillo-Jaramillo, C., Charro-Salgado, A., Perez-Infante, V., Lopez del Campo, G., Botella-Llusia, J., Coy, D.H., and Schally, A.V., Clinical studies with D-Trp^{6}-luteinizing hormone-releasing hormone in anovulatory women, Fertil. Steril., 29, 418, 1978.

34. Wentz, A.C., Clinical applications of luteinizing hormone-releasing hormone, Fertil. Steril., 28, 901, 1977.

35. Schneider, H.P.G., Diagnostic and therapeutic use of luteinizing hormone-releasing hormone (LH-RH), Arch. Pharmacol., 297, S71, 1977.

36. Cantor, B., Kalra, P.S., Buhi, W.C., Birk, S.A., Spellacy, W.N., Factors influencing the dynamics of gonadotropin response following bolus infusion of luteinizing hormone-releasing factor in women with menstrual abnormalities, Fertil. Steril., 28, 526, 1977.

37. Wentz, A.C., and Jones, G.S., Prognosis in primary amenorrhea, Fertil. Steril., 29, 614, 1978.

38. Böhm, P., Fenske, M., Häffele, R., and König, A., Limited significance of the LRH test in the diagnosis of ovarian dysfunction, Acta Endocrinol., 89, 438, 1978.

39. Dericks-Tan, J.S.E., Hammer, E., and Taubert, H.-D., The effect of D-Ser $(TBU)^6$-LH-RH-EA^{10} upon gonadotropin release in normally cyclic women, J. Clin. Endocrinol. Metab., 45, 597, 1977.

40. Corbin, A., Beattie, C.W., Jones, R., and Bex, F., Peptide contraception: Antifertility properties of LH-RH analogues, Int. J. Gynaecol. Obstet., 16, 359, 1979.

41. Nillius, S.J., Bergquist, C., and Wide, L., Inhibition of ovulation in women by chronic treatment with a stimulatory LRH analogue - a new approach to birth control?, Contraception, 17, 537, 1978.

42. Koyama, T., Ohkura, T., Kumasaka, T., and Saito, M., Effect of post-ovulatory treatment with a luteinizing hormone-releasing hormone analog on the plasma level of progesterone in women, Fertil. Steril., 30, 549, 1978.

43. Lemay, A., Labrie, F., Ferland, L., and Raynaud, J., Possible luteolytic effects of luteinizing hormone-releasing hormone in normal women, Fertil. Steril., 31, 29, 1979.

44. Casper, R.F., and Yen, S.S.C., Induction of luteolysis in the human with a long-acting analog of luteinizing hormone-releasing factor, Science, 205, 408, 1979.

45. Bergquist, C., Nillius, S.J., and Wide, L., Inhibition of ovulation in women by intranasal treatment with a luteinizing hormone-releasing hormone agonist, Contraception, 19, 497, 1979.

46. Crosignani, P.G., Trojsi, L., Attanasio, A., Tonani, E., and Donini, P., Hormonal profiles in anovulatory patients treated with gonadotropins and synthetic luteinizing hormone releasing hormone, Obstet. Gynecol., 46, 15, 1975.

47. Nillius, S.J., and Wide, L., Gonadotrophin-releasing hormone treatment for induction of follicular maturation and ovulation in amenorrhoeic women with anorexia nervosa, Br. Med. J., 3, 405, 1975.

48. Grimes, E.M., Taymor, M.L., and Thompson, I.E., Induction of timed ovulation with synthetic luteinizing hormone-releasing hormone in women undergoing insemination therapy. I. Effect of a single parenteral administration at midcycle, Fertil. Steril., 26, 277, 1975.

49. Zarate, A., Valdes-Vallina, F., Gonzalez, A., Perez-Ubierna, C., Canales, E.S., and Schally, A.V., Therapeutic effect of synthetic luteinizing hormone-releasing hormone (LH-RH) in male infertility due to idiopathic azoospermia and oligospermia, Fertil. Steril., 24, 485, 1973.

50. Mortimer, C.H., McNeilly, A.S., Fisher, R.A., Murray, M.A.F., Besser, G.M., Gonadotropin-releasing hormone therapy in hypogonadal males with hypothalamic or pituitary dysfunction, Br. Med. J., 4, 617, 1974.

51. Schwarzstein, L., Aparicio, N.J., Turner, D., Calamera, J.C., Mancini, R., and Schally, A.V., Use of synthetic luteinizing hormone-releasing hormone in treatment of oligospermic men: a preliminary report, Fertil. Steril., 26, 331, 1975.

52. Aparicio, N.J., Schwarzstein, L., Turner, E.A., Turner, D., Mancini, R., and Schally, A.V., Treatment of idiopathic normogonadotropic oligoastheno-

spermia with synthetic luteinizing hormone-releasing hormone, Fertil. Steril., 27, 549, 1976.

53. Tharandt, L., Schulte, H., Benker, G., Hackenberg, K., and Reinwein, D., Treatment of isolated gonadotrophin deficiency in men with a more potent analogue of LH-RH, Horm. Metab. Res., 9, 342, 1977.

54. Tharandt, L., Schulte, H., Benker, G., Hackenberg, K., and Reinwein, D., Treatment of isolated gonadotrophin deficiency in men with synthetic LH-RH and a more potent analogue of LH-RH, Neuroendocrinology, 24, 195, 1977.

55. Smith, R., Donald, A., Espiner, E.A., and Stronach, S., The effects of prolonged administration of D-Ser(TBU)^6-LH-RH-EA^{10}(HOE 766) in subjects with hypogonadotrophic hypogonadism, Clin. Endocrinol., 11, 553, 1979.

56. Jaramillo-Jaramillo, C., Charro-Salgado, A.L., Perez-Infante, V., Obanza, E.B., Iglesias, F.C., Fernandez-Cruz, A., Coy, D.H., and Schally, A.V., Clinical studies with D-Trp^6-luteinizing hormone-releasing hormone in men with hypogonadotropic hypogonadism, Fertil. Steril., 30, 430, 1978.

57. Wiegelmann, W., Solbach, H.G., Kley, H.K., and Krüskemper, H.L., LH and FSH response to long-term application of an LHRH analog in normal males, Horm. Metab. Res., 9, 521, 1977.

58. Smith, R., Donald, R.A., Espiner, E.A., Stronach, S.G., and Edwards, I.A., Normal adults and subjects with hypogonadotrophic hypogonadism respond differently to D-Ser(TBU)^6-LH-RH-EA^{10}, J. Endocrinol. Metab., 48, 167, 1979.

59. Bergquist, C., Nillius, S.J., Bergh, T., Skarin, G., and Wide, L., Inhibitory effects on gonadotrophin secretion and gonadal function in men during chronic treatment with a potent stimulatory luteinizing hormone releasing hormone analogue, Acta Endocrinol., 91, 601, 1979.

60. Bartsch, G., and Frick, J., Therapeutic effects of luteinizing hormone releasing hormone (LH-RH) in cryptorchidism, Andrologia, 6, 197, 1974.

61. Happ, J., Weber, T., Callensee, W., Ermert, J.A., Eshkol, A., and Beyer, J., Treatment of cryptorchidism with a potent analog of gonadotropin-releasing hormone, Fertil. Steril., 29, 552, 1978.

62. Happ, J., Kollmann, F., Krawehl, C., Neubauer, M., Krause, U., Demisch, K., Sandow, J., Von Rechenberg, W., and Beyer, J., Treatment of cryptorchidism with pernasal gonadotropin-releasing hormone therapy, Fertil. Steril., 29, 546, 1978.

63. Guillemin, R., Amoss, M., Blackwell, R., Burgus, R., Grant, G., Ling, N., Monahan, M., Rivier, J., and Vale, W., Polypeptide antagonists of the hypothalamic luteinizing hormone-releasing factors, J. Reprod. Fertil., Suppl. 18, 23, 1973.

64. Fujino, M., Kobayashi, S., Obayashi, M., Shinagawa, S., Fukuda, T., Kitada, C., Nakayama, R., Yamazaki, I., White, W.F., and Rippel, R.H., Structure-activity relationships in the C-terminal part of luteinizing hormone releasing hormone (LH-RH), Biochem. Biophys. Res. Commun., 49, 863, 1972.

65. Coy, D.H., Vilchez-Martinez, J.A., Coy, E.J., Arimura, A., and Schally, A.V., A peptide inhibitor of luteinizing hormone-releasing hormone (LH-RH), J. Clin. Endocrinol. Metab., 37, 331, 1973.

66. Monahan, M., Amoss, M., Anderson, H., and Vale, W., Synthetic analogs of the hypothalamic luteinizing hormone releasing factor with increased agonist or antagonist properties, Biochemistry, 12, 4616, 1973.

67. Rees, R.W.A., Foell, T.J., Chai, S.-Y., and Grant, N., Synthesis and biological activities of analogs of the luteinizing hormone-releasing hormone (LH-RH) modified in position 2, J. Med. Chem., 17, 1016, 1974.

68. Yardley, J.P., Foell, T.J., Beattie, C.W., and Grant, N.H., Antagonism of luteinizing hormone release and of ovulation by an analog of the

luteinizing hormone-releasing hormone, J. Med. Chem., 18, 1244, 1975.

69. Humphries, J., Fisher, G., Wan, Y.-P., Folkers, K., and Bowers, C.Y., Analogs of the luteinizing hormone-releasing hormone to study conformational aspects of the aromatic amino acid moieties and inhibition, J. Med. Chem., 17, 569, 1974.

70. Vilchez-Martinez, J.A., Schally, A.V., Coy, D.H., Coy, E.J., Debeljuk, L., and Arimura, A., In vivo inhibition of LH release by a synthetic antagonist of LH-releasing hormone (LH-RH), Endocrinology, 95, 213, 1974.

71. Coy, D.H., Coy, E.J., Schally, A.V., Vilchez-Martinez, J.A., Debeljuk, L., Carter, W.H., and Arimura, A., Stimulatory and inhibitory analogs of luteinizing hormone releasing hormone, Biochemistry, 13, 323, 1974.

72. Vilchez-Martinez, J.A., Schally, A.V., Debeljuk, L., Coy, D.H., Coy, E.J., Arimura, A., and Yanaihara, N., Development of a method to test anti-LH-RH activity in rats, Neuroendocrinology, 14, 121, 1974.

73. Humphries, J., Wan, Y.-P., Folkers, K., and Bowers, C.Y., On the importance of position one of ovulation inhibitors, as based on studies on [D-Phe^2,Pro^3,D-Phe^6]-LHRH, Biochem. Biophys. Res. Commun., 78, 506, 1977.

74. Humphries, J., Wan, Y.-P., Folkers, K., and Bowers, C.Y., Inhibitory analogues of the luteinizing hormone-releasing hormone having D-aromatic residues in positions 2 and 6 and variation in position 3, J. Med. Chem., 21, 120, 1978.

75. Grieg, F., and Weisz, J., Preovulatory levels of luteinizing hormone, the critical period and ovulation in rats, J. Endocrinol., 57, 235, 1973.

76. Coy, D.H., Schally, A.V., Vilchez-Martinez, J.A., Coy, E.J., and Arimura, A., Stimulatory and inhibitory analogs of LH-RH, in Hypothalamic Hormones: Chemistry, Physiology, Pharmacology and Clinical Uses, Motta, M.,

Crosignani, P.G., and Martini, L., Eds., Academic, New York, 1975, 1.

77. De la Cruz, A., Coy, D.H., Schally, A.V., Coy, E.J., De la Cruz, K.G., and Arimura, A., Blockade of the preovulatory LH surge in hamsters by an inhibitory analog of LH-RH, Proc. Soc. Exp. Biol. Med., 149, 576, 1975.

78. Corbin, A., and Beattie, C.W., Inhibition of the pre-ovulatory proestrous gonadotropin surge, ovulation and pregnancy with a peptide analogue of luteinizing hormone releasing hormone, Endocr. Res. Commun., 2, 1, 1975.

79. Beattie, C.W., Corbin, A., Foell, T.J., Garsky, V., McKinley, W.A., Rees, R.W.A., Sarantakis, D., and Yardley, J.P., Luteinizing hormone-releasing hormone: Antiovulatory activity of analogs substituted in positions 2 and 6, J. Med. Chem., 18, 1247, 1975.

80. Beattie, C.W., Corbin, A., Foell, T.J., Garsky, V., Rees, R.W.A., and Yardley, J., Anti-ovulatory/anti-pregnancy effects of [D-Phe^2]-LRH analogs administered early in the rat estrous cycle, Contraception, 13, 341, 1976.

81. Corbin, A., and Beattie, C.W., Effect of luteinizing hormone releasing hormone (LHRH) and an LHRH antagonist on hypothalamic and plasma LHRH of hypophysectomized rats, Endocrinology, 98, 247, 1976.

82. De la Cruz, A., Coy, D.H., Vilchez-Martinez, J.A., Arimura, A., and Schally, A.V., Blockade of ovulation in rats by inhibitory analogs of luteinizing hormone-releasing hormone, Science, 191, 195, 1976.

83. Humphries, J., Wan, Y.-P., Folkers, K., and Bowers, C.Y., Inhibition of the activity of the luteinizing hormone-releasing hormone (LH-RH) by analogues with variations at positions 2, 3, and 6 and the carboxy terminus, J. Med. Chem., 20, 967, 1977.

84. Wan, Y.-P., Humphries, J., Fisher, G., Folkers, K., and Bowers, C.Y., Inhibitors of the luteinizing hormone-releasing hormone based upon modifications in the 2, 3, and 6 positions. J. Med. Chem., 19, 199, 1976.

85. Humphries, J., Wan, J.-R., Folkers, K., and Bowers, C.Y., Presence of proline in position 3 for potent inhibition of the activity of the luteinizing hormone-releasing hormone and of ovulation, Biochem. Biophys. Res. Commun., 72, 939, 1976.

86. Pedroza, E., Vilchez-Martinez, J.A., Coy, D.H., Arimura, A., and Schally, A.V., Correlation between in vivo inhibition of gonadotropin release induced by LH-RH and the blockade of ovulation by synthetic analogues of LH-RH, Int. J. Fertil., 23, 294, 1978.

87. Bowers, C.Y., and Folkers, K., Contraception and inhibition of ovulation by minipump infusion of the luteinizing hormone releasing hormone, active analogues and antagonists, Biochem. Biophys. Res. Commun., 72, 1003, 1976.

88. Humphries, J., Wasiak, T., Wan, Y.-P., and Folkers, K., An antiovulatory decapeptide of higher potency which has an L-amino acid (Ac-Pro) in position 1, Biochem. Biophys. Res. Commun., 85, 709, 1978.

89. Rivier, J.E., and Vale, W.W., [D-pGlu^{1},D-Phe^{2},D-Trp^{3,6}]-LRF. A potent luteinizing hormone releasing factor antagonist in vitro and inhibitor of ovulation in the rat, Life Sci., 23, 869, 1978.

90. Rivier, C., Rivier, J., and Vale, W., Effect of the LRF-antagonist [D-pGlu^{1},D-Phe^{2},D-Trp^{3,6}]-LRF on pregnancy in the rat, Contraception, 19, 185, 1979.

91. Wasiak, T., Humphries, J., Folkers, K., and Bowers, C.Y., A new category of ovulation inhibitors linear LH-RH analogues having more than ten residues, Biochem. Biophys. Res. Commun., 86, 843, 1979.

92. Seprodi, J., Coy, D.H., Vilchez-Martinez, J.A., Pedroza, E., and Schally, A.V., Branched-chain analogues of luteinizing hormone-releasing hormone, J. Med. Chem., 21, 276, 1978.

92a. Bowers, C.Y., Humphries, J., Wasiak, T., Folkers, K., Reynolds, G.A., and Reichert, L.E. Jr., On the inhibitory effects of luteinizing hormone-releasing hormone analogs, Endocrinology, 106, 674, 1980.

93. Hagino, N., Coy, D.H., Schally, A.V., and Arimura, A., Inhibition of

release in the baboon by inhibitory analogs of luteinizing hormone releasing hormone, Horm. Metab. Res., 9, 247, 1977.

94. Gosselin, R.E., Fuller, G.B., Coy, D.H., Schally, A.V., and Hobson, W.C., Inhibition of gonadotropin release in chimpanzees by the LH-RH antagonist ($D-Phe^2,D-Trp^3,D-Phe^6$)-LH-RH, Proc. Soc. Exp. Biol. Med., 161, 21, 1979.

95. Corbin, A., Jaszczak, S., Peluso, J., Shandilya, N.L., and Hafez, E.S.E., Effect of LH-RH peptide antagonist on serum LH, ovulation and menstrual cycle of crab-eating macaque, Contraception, 18, 105, 1978.

96. Gonzalez-Barcena, D., Kastin, A.J., Coy, D.H., Nikolics, K., and Schally, A.V., Suppression of gonadotrophin release in man by an inhibitory analogue of LH-releasing hormone, Lancet, 2, 997, 1977.

97. Banik, U.K., and Givner, M.L., Ovulation induction and antifertility effects of an LH-RH analogue (AY-25,205) in cyclic rats, J. Reprod. Fertil., 44, 87, 1975.

98. Banik, U.K., and Givner, M.L., Effects of a luteinizing hormone-releasing hormone analog on mating and fertility in rats, Fertil. Steril., 27, 1078, 1976.

99. Corbin, A., and Beattie, C.W., Regulation of female mammalian fertility with luteinizing hormone releasing hormone (LRH) and related analogues, in Ovulation in the Human, Crosignani, P.G., and Mishell, D.R., Eds., Academic, New York, 1976, 193.

100. Corbin, A., and Beattie, C.W., Post-coital contraceptive and uterotrophic effects of luteinizing hormone releasing hormone, Endocr. Res. Commun., 2, 445, 1975.

101. Coy, D.H., Labrie, F., Savary, M., Coy, E.J., and Schally, A.V., LH-releasing activity of potent LH-RH analogs in vitro, Biochem. Biophys. Res. Commun., 67, 576, 1975.

102. Vale, W., Rivier, C., Brown, M., Leppaluoto, J., Ling, N., Monahan, M., and Rivier, J., Pharmacology of hypothalamic regulatory peptides, Clin. Endocrinol., Suppl. 5, 261S, 1976.

103. Humphrey, R.R., Windsor, B.L., Bousley, F.G., and Edgren, R.A., Anti-fertility effects of an analog of luteinizing hormone releasing hormone (LHRH) in rats, Contraception, 14, 625, 1976.

104. Arimura, A., Pedroza, E., Vilchez-Martinez, J., and Schally, A.V., Prevention of implantation by [D-Trp^6]-LH-RH in the rat: Comparative study with the effects of large doses of HCG on pregnancy, Endocr. Res. Commun., 4, 357, 1977.

105. Corbin, A., Beattie, C.W., Rees, R.W.A., Yardley, J., Foell, T.J., Chai, S.Y., McGregor, H., Garsky, V., Sarantakis, D., and McKinley, W.A., Post-coital contraceptive effects of agonist analogs of luteinizing hormone-releasing hormone, Fertil. Steril., 28, 471, 1977.

106. Corbin, A., Beattie, C.W., Tracy, J., Jones, R., Foell, T.J., Yardley, J., and Rees, R.W.A., The anti-reproductive pharmacology of LH-RH and agonistic analogues, Int. J. Fertil., 23, 81, 1978.

107. Corbin, A., Bex, F.J., Yardley, J.P., Rees, R.W.A., Foell, T.J., and Sarantakis, D., Agonist (ovulation induction) and post-coital contraceptive properties of [D-Ala^6] and [D-Trp^6]-LHRH series, Endocr. Res. Commun. 6, 1, 1979.

108. Corbin, A., Beattie, C.W., Yardley, J., and Foell, T.J., Post-coital contraceptive effects of an agonistic analogue of luteinizing hormone releasing hormone, Endocr. Res. Commun., 3, 359, 1976.

109. Rippel, R.H., and Johnson, E.S., Regression of corpora lutea in the rabbit after injection of a gonadotropin-releasing peptide, Proc. Soc. Biol. Med., 152, 29, 1976.

110. Hilliard, J., Pang, C.N., and Sawyer, C.H., Effects of luteinizing hormone releasing hormone on fetal survival in pregnant rabbits, Fertil. Steril., 27, 421, 1976.

111. Windsor, B.L., Humphrey, R.R., Reel, J.R., and Edgren, R.A., Postnidatory effects of luteinizing hormone releasing hormone (LHRH) in hamsters, Int. J. Fertil., 22, 184, 1977.

112. Beattie, C.W., and Corbin, A., Pre- and post-coital contraceptive activity of LH-RH in the rat, Biol. Reprod., 16, 333, 1977.

113. Johnson, E.S., Gendrich, R.L., and White, W.F., Delay of puberty and inhibition of reproductive processes in the rat by a gonadotropin-releasing hormone agonist analog, Fertil. Steril., 27, 853, 1976.

114. Rippel, R.H., and Johnson, E.S., Inhibition of HCG-induced ovarian and uterine weight augmentation in the immature rat by analogs of GnRH, Proc. Soc. Exp. Biol. Med., 152, 432, 1976.

115. Vilchez-Martinez, J.A., Pedroza, E., Arimura, A., and Schally, A.V., Paradoxical effects of D-Trp^6-Luteinizing hormone-releasing hormone on the hypothalamic pituitary-gonadal axis in immature female rats, Fertil. Steril., 31, 677, 1979.

116. Richards, J.S., Ireland, J.J., Rao, M.C., Bernath, G.A., Midgley, A.R., Jr., and Reichert, L.E., Jr., Ovarian follicular development in the rat: Hormone receptor regulation by estradiol, follicle stimulating hormone and luteinizing hormone, Endocrinology, 99, 1562, 1976.

117. Rao, M.C., Richards, J.S., Midgley, A.R., Jr., and Reichert, L.E., Jr., Regulation of gonadotropin receptors by luteinizing hormone in granulosa cells, Endocrinology, 101, 512, 1977.

118. Bex, F.J., and Corbin, A., Mechanism of the postcoital contraceptive effect of luteinizing hormone-releasing hormone: Ovarian luteinizing

hormone receptor interactions, Endocrinology, 105, 139, 1979.

119. Kledzik, G.S., Cusan, L., Auclair, C., Kelly, P.A., and Labrie, F., Inhibitory effect of a luteinizing hormone (LH)-releasing hormone agonist on rat ovarian LH and follicle-stimulating hormone receptor levels during pregnancy, Fertil. Steril., 29, 560, 1978.

120. Kledzik, G.S., Cusan, L., Auclair, C., Kelly, P.A., and Labrie, F., Inhibition of ovarian luteinizing hormone (LH) and follicle-stimulating hormone receptor levels with an LH-releasing hormone agonist during the estrous cycle in the rat, Fertil. Steril., 30, 348, 1978.

121. Beattie, C.W., Corbin, A., Cole, G., Corry, S., Jones, R.C., Koch, K., and Tracy, J., Mechanism of the post-coital contraceptive effect of LH-RH in the rat. I. Serum hormone levels during chronic LH-RH administration, Biol. Reprod., 16, 322, 1977.

122. Yoshinaga, K., Effect of an LHRH analog on the pituitary function of pregnant rats, Abstract 495, Program of the 60th Annual Meeting of the Endocrine Society, Miami, 1978.

123. Humphrey, R.R., Windsor, B.L., Reel, J.R., and Edgren, R.A., The effects of luteinizing hormone (LHRH) in pregnant rats. I. Postnidatory effects, Biol. Reprod., 16, 614, 1977.

124. Cusan, L., Auclair, C., Belanger, A., Ferland, L., Kelly, P.A., Seguin, C., and Labrie, F., Inhibitory effects of long-term treatment with a luteinizing hormone-releasing hormone agonist on the pituitary-gonadal axis in male and female rats, Endocrinology, 104, 1369, 1979.

125. Pencharz, R.I., and Long, J.A., Hypophysectomy in the pregnant rat, Am. J. Anat., 53, 117, 1933.

126. Pepe, G., and Rothchild, I., The effect of hypophysectomy on day 12 of pregnancy on the serum progesterone level and time of parturition in the

rat, Endocrinology, 91, 1380, 1972.

127. Macdonald, G.J., and Beattie, C.W., Pregnancy failure in hypophysectomized rats following LH-RH administration, Life Sci., 24, 1103, 1979.

128. Bex, F.J., and Corbin, A., LHRH or LHRH agonist-induced termination of pregnancy in hypophysectomized (HYPX) rats: Extrapituitary site of action, Abstract 436, Program of the 61st Annual Meeting of the Endocrine Society, Anaheim, 1979.

129. Khodr, G.S., and Siler-Khodr, T., Localization of luteinizing hormone-releasing factor in the human placenta, Fertil. Steril., 29, 523, 1978.

130. Khodr, G.S., and Siler-Khodr, T., The effect of luteinizing hormone-releasing factor on human chorionic gonadotropin secretion, Fertil. Steril., 30, 301, 1978.

131. Siler-Khodr, T.M., and Khodr, G.S., Content of luteinizing hormone-releasing factor in the human placenta, Am. J. Obstet. Gynecol., 130, 216, 1978.

132. Haour, F., Tell, G., and Sanchez, P., Mise en evidence et dosage d'une gonadotrophine chorionique chez le rat (rCG), CR Acad. Sci. (Paris), 282, 1183, 1976.

133. Gibori, G., Antczak, E., and Rothchild, I., The role of estrogen in the regulation of luteal progesterone secretion in the rat after day 12 of pregnancy, Endocrinology, 100, 1483, 1977.

134. Gibori, G., and Keyes, P.L., Role of intraluteal estrogen in the regulation of the rat corpus luteum during pregnancy, Endocrinology, 102, 1176, 1978.

135. Mayar, M.Q., Tarnavsky, G.K., and Reeves, J.J., Ovarian growth and uptake of iodinated D-leu, des-Gly-NH_2^{10}-LHRH ethylamide in HCG treated rats, Proc. Soc. Exp. Biol. Med., 161, 216, 1979.

136. Hsueh, A.J.W., and Erickson, G.F., Extrapituitary action of gonadotropin-releasing hormone: Direct inhibition of ovarian steroidogenesis, Science, 204, 854, 1979.

137. Clayton, R.N., Harwood, J.P., and Catt, K.J., Gonadotropin-releasing hormone binds to luteal cells and inhibits progesterone production, Nature, 282, 90, 1979.

138. Ying, S., and Guillemin, R., (D-Trp^6-Pro^9-NEt)-luteinizing hormone-releasing factor inhibits follicular development in hypophysectomized rats, Nature, 280, 593, 1979.

138a. Jones, R.C., Local antifertility effect of luteinizing hormone-releasing hormone (LRH), Contraception, 20, 569, 1979.

139. Bex, F.J., and Corbin, A., Antifertility effects of LHRH and its agonists, in Reproductive Processes and Contraception, McKerns, K.W., Ed., Plenum, New York, 1980, in press.

140. Lemay, A., Labrie, F., and Raynaud, J.P., Luteolytic activity of LHRH and [D-Ser(TBu)^6,Des-Gly-NH_2^{10}]LHRH ethylamide: A new and physiological approach to contraception in women, in Proceedings from the International Symposium on Basic and Clinical Aspects of LH-RH and Analogues in Fertility Regulation, Int. J. Fertil., 1980, in press.

141. Bergquist, C., Nillius, S.J., and Wide, L., Intranasal gonadotropin-releasing hormone agonist as a contraceptive agent, Lancet, 2, 215, 1979.

142. Hsueh, A.J., Dufau, M.L., and Catt, K.J., Regulation of luteinizing hormone receptors in testicular interstitial cells by gonadotropin, Biochem. Biophys. Res. Commun., 72, 1145, 1976.

143. Sharpe, R.M., hCG-induced decrease in availability of rat testes receptors, Nature, 264, 644, 1976.

144. Corbin, A., and Bex, F.J., Inhibition of male reproductive processes with an LHRH agonist, in Regulation of Male Fertility, Cunningham, G.R.,

Schill, W.B., and Hafez, E.S.E., Eds., Martinus Nyoff, The Hague, The Netherlands, 1980, in press.

145. Auclair, C., Kelly, P.A., Labrie, F., Coy, D.H., and Schally, A.V., Inhibition of testicular luteinizing hormone receptor level by treatment with a potent luteinizing hormone-releasing hormone agonist or human chorionic gonadotropin, Biochem. Biophys. Res. Commun., 76, 855, 1977.

146. Auclair, C., Kelly, P.A., Coy, D.H., Schally, A.V., and Labrie, F., Potent inhibitory activity of [D-Leu^6,Des-Gly-NH_2^{10}] LHRH ethylamide on LH/hCG and PRL testicular receptor levels in the rat, Endocrinology, 101, 1890, 1977.

147. Bex, F.J., and Corbin, A., Inhibition of reproductive processes in the immature and mature male rat with an LHRH agonist, Abstract 6, Program 3rd Annual Meeting American Society of Andrology, Nashville, 1978.

148. Pelletier, G., Cusan, L., Auclair, C., Kelly, P.A., Desy, L., and Labrie, F., Inhibition of spermatogenesis in the rat by treatment with [D-Ala^6, Des-Gly_2^{10}] LHRH ethylamide, Endocrinology, 103, 641, 1978.

149. Rivier, C., Rivier, J., and Vale, W., Chronic effects of [D-Trp^6,Pro^9, NEt] luteinizing hormone-releasing factor on reproductive processes in the male rat, Endocrinology, 105, 1191, 1979.

150. Corbin, A., Contraception peptidique: Regulation de la fertilite par les analogues du LHRH, in Actualites Gynecologiques (9th Serie), Netter, A., and Gorins, A., Eds., Masson, Paris, 1978, 235.

151. Cusan, L., Auclair, C., Belanger, A., Ferland, L., Kelly, P.A., Seguin, C., and Labrie, F., Inhibitory effects of long-term treatment with an LHRH agonist on the pituitary-gonadal axis in male and female rats, Endocrinology, 104, 1369, 1979.

152. Oshima, H., Nankin, H., Fan, D.-F., Troen, P., Yanaihara, T., Nizato, N., Yoshida, K.-I., and Ochiai, K.-I., Delay in sexual maturation of rats caused by synthetic LH-releasing hromone: Enhancement of steroid Δ^4-5^α-hydrogenase in testes, Biol. Reprod., 12, 491, 1975.

153. Tcholakian, R.K., De la Cruz, A., Chowdhury, M., Steinberger, A., Coy, D.H., and Schally, A.V., Unusual anti-reproductive properties of the analog [D-Leu^6,Des-Gly-NH_2^{10}]-luteinizing hormone-releasing hormone ethylamide in male rats, Fertil. Steril., 30, 600, 1978.

154. Sharpe, R.M., Fraser, H.M., and Sandow, J., Effect of treatment with an agonist of luteinizing hormone-releasing hormone on early maturational changes in pituitary and testicular function in the rat, J. Endocrinol., 80, 249, 1979.

155. Sharpe, R.M., and Fraser, H.M., Inhibition of maturational changes in Leydig cell function after treatment of rats with an agonist of luteinizing hormone releasing hormone, J. Endocrinol., 81, 159, 1979.

156. Catt, K.J., Baukal, A.J., Davies, T.F., and Dufau, M.L., Luteinizing hormone-releasing hormone-induced regulation of gonadotropin and prolactin receptors in the rat testis, Endocrinology, 104, 17, 1979.

157. Sandow, J., Von Rechenberg, W., Jerzabek, G., and Stoll, W., Pituitary gonadotropin inhibition by a highly active analog of luteinizing hormone-releasing hormone, Fertil. Steril., 30, 205, 1978.

158. Hsueh, A.J.W., and Erickson, G.F., Extra-pituitary inhibition of testicular function by luteinizing hormone-releasing hormone, Nature, 281, 66, 1979.

159. Arimura, A., Serafini, P., Talbot, S., and Schally, A.V., Reduction of testicular luteinizing hormone/human chorionic gonadotropin receptors by [D-Trp^6]-luteinizing hormone releasing hormone in hypophysectomized rats, Biochem. Biophys. Res. Commun., 90, 687, 1979.

160. Seguin, C., Cusan, L., Belanger, A., Reeves, J.J., Kelly, P.A., and Labrie, F., Direct effects of LHRH agonists on the rat testis, Program 5th Annual Meeting American Society of Andrology, Chicago, 1980.

161. Badger, T.M., Beitins, I.Z., Ostrea, T., Crisafulli, J., Little, R., and Saidel, M., Effects of luteinizing hormone releasing hormone and one of its highly potent analogs ($D-Trp^6-Pro^9$-NHEt-LRF) on in vitro testosterone synthesis, Abstract 430, Program of the 61st Annual Meeting of the Endocrine Society, Anaheim, 1979.

162. Belanger, A., Auclair, C., and Caron, S., Role of prolactin in the LHRH agonist-induced blockage of testicular steroidogenesis, Abstract 717, Program of the 61st Annual Meeting of the Endocrine Society, Anaheim, 1979.

163. Belanger, A., Auclair, C., and Caron, S., Inhibition of the testicular steroidogenic pathway by treatment with an LHRH agonist in the rat, Abstract 93, Program of 12th Annual Meeting of the Society for the Study of Reproduction, Quebec, 1979.

164. Rivier, J.E., and Vale, W.W., Hormonal secretion in male rats chronically treated with [$D-Trp^6, Pro^9$-NHEt]-LRF, Life Sci., 25, 1065, 1979.

165. Flickinger, C.J., The influence of progestin and androgen on the fine structure of the male reproductive tract of the rat, Anat. Rec. 187, 405, 1977.

166. Hemm, R.D., Pollock, J.J., Arslanoglou, L., Authier, L., Preclinical safety studies of a synthetic gonadotrophin releasing hormone (LH-RH), Toxicol. Appl. Pharmacol., 29, 99, 1974.

167. Sandow, J., Rechenberg, W.V., and Jerzabek, G., Pharmacological effects of chronic treatment with the LH-RH analogue $D-Ser(TBu)^6$ ethylamide,

Acta Endocrinol., Suppl. 208, 33, 1977.

168. Hemm, R.D., Arslanoglou, L., and Pollock, J.J., Comparative teratogenicity studies of a synthetic gonadotrophin releasing hormone, Teratology, 9, A19, 1974.

169. Ayerst Brochure, HRF (Gonadorelin LH/FSH/RH): A diagnostic aid for assessing pituitary function, Ayerst International, 1974.

170. Sandow, J., Von Rechenberg, W., Konig, W., Hahn, M., Jerzabek, G., and Fraser, H., Physiological studies with highly active analogues of LH-RH, in Hypothalamic Hormones - Chemistry, Physiology, and Clinical Applications, Gupta, D., and Voelter, W., Eds., Verlag Chemie, Weinheim, 1978, 307.

171. Sandow, J., Toxicological evaluation of drugs affecting the hypothalamic-pituitary system, Pharmc. Ther., 5, 297, 1979.

INDEX

Chapter 1

Aldosterone 3f, 31f, 38
Angiotensin I 5, 12f, 31f
Angiotensin II 3f, 12f, 32f
Angiotensin III 5, 7
Angiotensin Converting Enzyme 3f, 8f, 12f, 33f
Angiotensinogen 5
Arterial Wall Renin 35
Bothropos Jararaca 8
Bradykinin 5, 7f, 31f, 36
BPP_{9a} 9
Capoten
Captopril 3, 9f
Chronic Renal Failure
Congestive Heart Failure 32f
DOCA-Salt Hypertensive Rats 24
Essential Hypertension 3, 16f, 24f
Hemorrhagic Shock 33
Hydralazine 17, 21
Hypertension 11, 16f, 33f, 39
Kallidin 5, 8
Kallikrein 3f, 7f, 31
1-Kidney, 1-Clip Renal Hypertensive Rats (1K-RHR) 19f, 31
2-Kidney, 1-Clip Renal Hypertensive Rats (2K-RHR) 16f, 31, 34, 35, 39
Kinin 3f, 31
Kininase 5, 7f
Kininogens 7f
Prostaglandin 3f, 14, 38
Renin 3f, 24f, 30f, 35
Renovascular Hypertension 6f, 24f
Saralasin 34
Spontaneously Hypertensive Rats (SHR) 21f, 34
SQ 14,225 11
SQ 20,881 35
Teprotide 3, 9f, 19, 21, 32
Zinc 5, 11

Chapter 2

Somatostatin 56-97 inclusive
- Analogues 93f
  - Duration of Activity 93f
  - Molecular Configuration 93f
  - Potency 94f
  - Selectivity 94f
  - Synthetic Approach 96f
- Effects on:
  - ACTH 62
  - Behavior 58
  - Blood; Blood Clotting 65
  - Calcitonin 62
  - Cardiovascular Function 65
  - FSH 62
  - Gastrointestinal Function 63f
  - Glucagon 63, 65f
  - Glucose 68f
  - Glycerol 72
  - Growth Hormone (GH) 56, 61
  - Insulin 65f
  - Ketone Body Levels 69f, 72
  - Lactate Levels, Plasma 72
  - LH 62
  - Nervous System 60f
  - Parathyroid Hormone 62
  - Posterior Pituitary Hormones 61
  - Prolactin 62
  - Renal Function 64f
  - Thyroid 62f
  - TSH 61f
- Mechanism of Action
  - Calcium Mediation 73f
  - Cyclic Nucleotide Metabolism 73f
  - Membrane Binding 73
  - Protein Synthesis 72
- Metabolism
  - Half-Life 77
  - Inactivation, Sites of 77
  - Degradation 77
- Physiological Role
  - Neurohormones 77f
  - Neurotransmitters 77f
  - Parahormones 78
- Secretory Control
  - Acetylcholine 84
  - Amino Acid Substrates 81
  - Calcium Modulation 83
  - Catecholamines 83f
  - Glucose Stimulation 79f
  - Monoamines 83f

Opioids 86
Pancreatic D Cells 63, 87
Peptide Hormones 86f
Serotonin 84
Therapeutic Use
Diabetes 87, 89f
Hypoglycemia, Reactive 90
Ulcers 90
Tissue Distribution 58f

Chapter 3

Fertility regulating botanicals
Animal species in which investigated/ in which effects of, reported,
Bat 186
Cattle 175, 196
Dog 171, 186
Gerbil 186
Guinea pig 171, 175-176
Hamster 160, 169
Human 156, 169, 171-185, 189-192, 197
Monkey 157, 175-178, 191
Mouse 159-160, 166, 168-169, 175, 177-179, 185-186, 196
Rabbit 154, 160, 168-169, 171-178, 191
Rat 155-156, 160-169, 171-175, 179-187, 191-193
Sheep 151-155, 175
Swine 196
Compounds investigated for/ reported as having,
Antifertility effects in females,
Aristolic acid 160
Aristolic acid methyl ester 160
Colchicine 169
p-Coumaric acid 160
Daturalactone 160
Desacetylmethylcolchicine 168-169
Embelin 163, 165
Maytansine 169
Miroestrol 155-156
Podophyllotoxin 168
Vinblastine 168-169
Vincristine 169
Zearalenone 196
See also: Fertility regulating botanicals, compounds investigated for/reported as having, uterine stimulant activity
See also: Plants, estrogenic
Antifertility effects in males,
Colchicine 197
Gossypol 189-193
Gossypol acetic acid 191
Vinblastine 185-186
Vincristine 185-186
m-Xylohydroquinone 189
Zearalenone 196
Spermicidal activity,
Lebbekanin-E (see Table 3) 180-181
Lemmatoxin 182
Lemmatoxin-C 182
Oleanoglycotoxin-A 182
Samanin-D 184
Scheffleroside 182
See also: Table 3 (pp 180-181)
Uterine stimulant activity,
Albitocin 175
Leonurine 172
Montanol 176
Plumbagin 171
Serotonin 174
Trichosanthin 177-179
Zoapatanol 176
Plant species investigated for/reported as having,
Antifertility effects in females,
Aristolochia indica 159-160
Aristolochia triangularis 169
Butea monosperma (Butea frondosa) 163
Claviceps purpurea (ergot) 170, 196
Cuminum oyminum 167
Curcuma longa 167
Datura quercifolia 160
Daucus carota 167
Embelia ribes 163-166
Hibiscus rosa-sinensis 162-163
Hyptis suaveolens 167
Pinus ponderosa 196-197
Pueraria mirifica 155-156
Pueraria tuberosa 156

See also: Fertility regulating botanicals, plant species investigated for/reported as having, uterine stimulant activity
See also: Plants, estrogenic
Antifertility effects in males,
Aristolochia indica 186
Catharanthus rossus 185
Gossypium hirsutum 189
Hibiscus rosa-sinensis 186-187
Malvaviscus conzattii 186
Momordica charantia 186
Pisum sativum 189
Spermicidal activity
Calendula officinalis 182
Phytolacca americana 182
Phytolacca dodecandra 182
Pithecellobium saman 184
Schefflera capitata 182
See also: Table 3 (pp 180-181)
Uterine stimulant activity
Albizia chinensis 175
Albizia grandibracteata 175
Albizia gummifera 175
Gloriosa superba 171
Leonurus artemisia 172
Montanoa tomentosa 176
Oldenlandia affinis 172-174
Plumbago zeylanica 171
Trichosanthes kirilowii 176-179
Plants,
Abortifacient 169-179
Antiovulatory 157
Antispermatogenic 184-193
Estrogenic 151-156
Interceptive 157-169
Spermicidal 179, 180-182, 184
See also: Fertility regulating botanicals

Chapter 4

Conceptive Effects 229f
Contraceptive, LHRH and Analogues as 236f, 259f
Downregulation of Gonadal Steroidogenic Function 253f,262,265
Estrogen Response 253
Extrapituitary (Direct Gonadal) Effect
Female 246f
Male 262f
Female Contraception 247f
Gonadotropin (LH and FSH) Inhibition 267
Gonadotropin (LH and FSH) Release 253f
Human Studies
Female 229f, 258f
Male 233f
Infertility, Treatment of
Female 229f
Male 233f
LHRH Agonists 228f, 246f, 260, 273f
LHRH Antagonists 228f, 235f, 273f
Luteolysis 232f
Male Contraception 262f, 269f
Mechanism of Anti-Reproductive Effect
Female 246f
Male 262f, 265f
Ovulation Induction 230f
Ovulation Inhibition 269
Paradoxical Antifertility Effects
Female 247f
Male 262f
Placental (rPL) Response 254
Pregnancy Termination
Claudogen Effect 247f
Interceptive Effect 247f
Progesterone Response 253
Prolactin Response 253
Reversibility of Antifertility Effect
Female 257f
Male 267f
Safety Studies
Preliminary Toxicology 270f
Secondary Pharmacology 270f
Spermatogenesis 263f
Synthesis of LHRH Analogues 236f
Testicular Function 235
Testosterone Response 263

GPSR Compliance

The European Union's (EU) General Product Safety Regulation (GPSR) is a set of rules that requires consumer products to be safe and our obligations to ensure this.

If you have any concerns about our products, you can contact us on ProductSafety@springernature.com

In case Publisher is established outside the EU, the EU authorized representative is:

Springer Nature Customer Service Center GmbH
Europaplatz 3
69115 Heidelberg, Germany

Batch number: 10584444

Printed by Printforce, the Netherlands